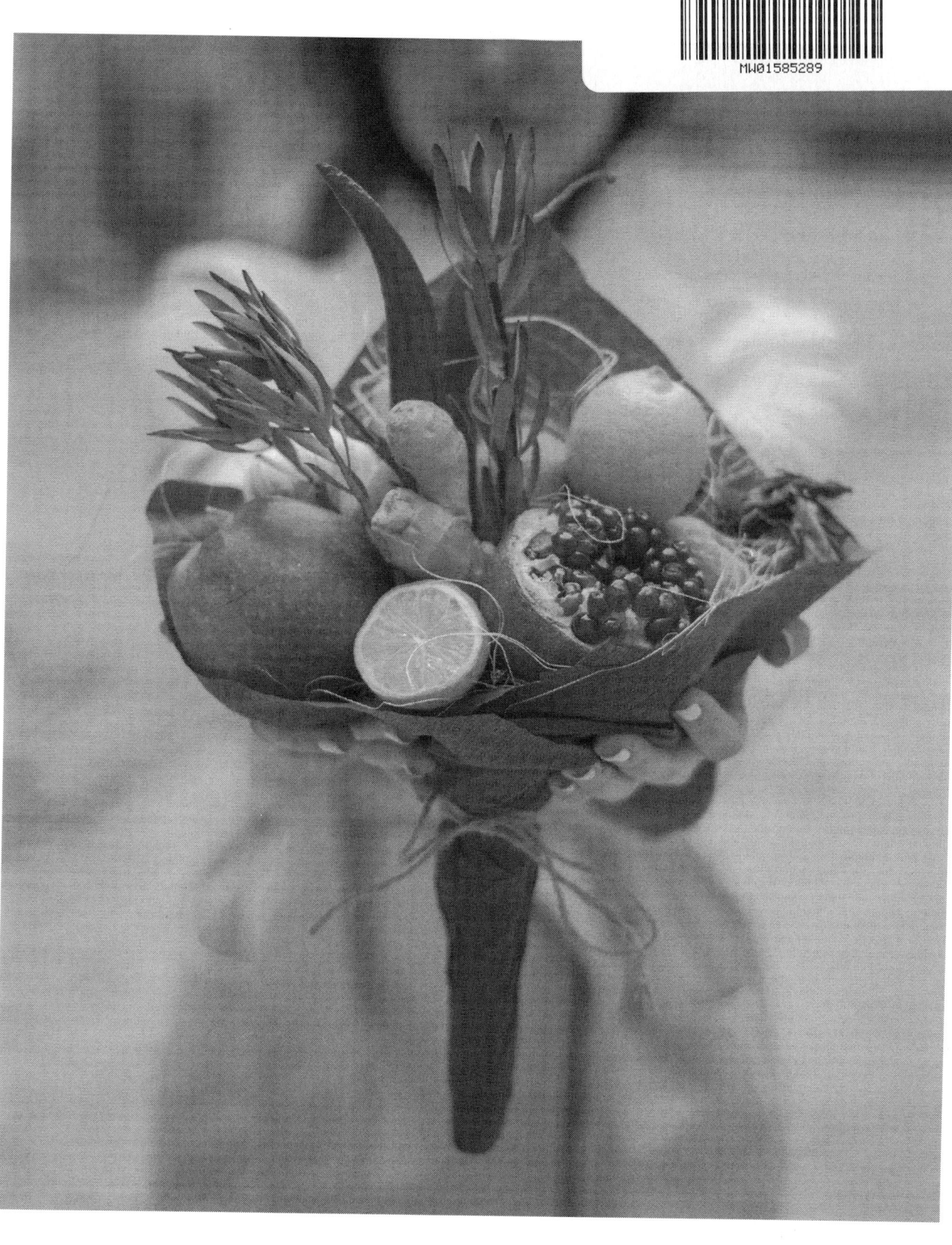

Table of Contents

INTRODUCTION 6
What is an Air Fryer? 6
Advantages of Using an Air Fryer 6
How an Air Fryer Works 7
How to Start Cooking in an Air Fryer 7
How to Clean and Maintain Your Air Fryer 8
Cooking Conversion Charts 9
    Mashed Potato Cakes 12
    Air Fried Spicy Potatoes 14
    Appealing Potato Kebabs 16
    Whole Baked Cauliflower 18
    Balsamic Cabbage Steaks 20
    Mouth-Melting Broccoli Bites 22
    Roasted Brussels Sprouts, Sweet Potatoes and Mushrooms 24
    Roasted Beetroots with Onion 26
    Turmeric Flavored Mashed Potato Stuffed Fritters 28
    Crispy Onion Pakoras 30
    Spring Onion and Cabbage Filled Wontons 32
    Crispy Masala Tofu 34
    Rosemary Zest Roasted Potatoes 36
    Bottle Gourd and Split Gram Patties 38
    Sweet Potato Garlic Chips 40
    Soya Sauce and Pepper Flavored Cauliflower 42
    Turmeric Zest Potato and Cauliflower 44
    Coriander and Chili Bites 46
    Mixed Herb Fried Potatoes 48
    Crunchy Zucchini Chips 50
    Grated Potato Fritters 52
    Masala Roasted Potato Wedges 54

- Roasted Peanuts 56
- Roasted Broccoli 58
- Air Fried Crispy Chili Bites 60
- Indian Style Kurkuri Lady Fingers 62
- Banana Wafers 64
- Baked Turnip Chips 66
- Air Fried Crusty Baked Tofu 68
- Roasted Cauliflower Bites 70
- Crunchy Cucumber Chips 72
- Roasted Potatoes, Brussels Sprouts, and Squash 74
- Fresh Bean Fries 76
- Baked Baisan Roti 78
- Dal Moong Pakoras 80
- Cinnamon Rolled Banana Bites 82
- Roasted Pineapples with Vanilla Zest 84
- Air Fryer Baked Apples 86

GIFT 88

As a thank you for purchasing this book,

I want to share with you a valuable GIFT!

You will find information about the gift at the end of the book.

Copyright 2018 by LESLEY LYNN HUDSON. © All rights reserved

All Rights Reserved. No part of this publication or the information in it may be quoted from or reproduced in any form by means such as printing, scanning, photocopying or otherwise without prior written permission of the copyright holder.

Disclaimer and Terms of Use: Effort has been made to ensure that the information in this book is accurate and complete, however, the author and the publisher do not warrant the accuracy of the information, text, and graphics contained within the book due to the rapidly changing nature of science, research, known and unknown facts and the internet.

All information is intended only to help you cooperate with your doctor, in your efforts toward desirable weight levels and health. Only your doctor can determine what is right for you. In addition to regular checkups and medical supervision, from your doctor, before starting any other weight loss program, you should consult with your personal physician.

The Author and the publisher do not hold any responsibility for errors, omissions or contrary interpretation of the subject matter herein. This book is presented solely for motivational and informational purposes only.

INTRODUCTION

What is an Air Fryer?

The air fryer is a recently introduced gadget which can be used for multiple purposes in the world of cooking. It has transformed cooking into a much easier and faster affair. In an air fryer, extremely hot air cooks food in a short period of time and in a healthier way. This is why an air fryer needs only a small amount of cooking oil, even though you're frying the food.

Advantages of Using an Air Fryer

- This novel technology has made it feasible to fry, roast, steam, bake, or grill any cuisine in one pot easily and without too much effort.
- Another chief advantage of this wonderful advanced equipment is only needing to use a small quantity of cooking oil as compared to any other types of fryers.
- An air fryer allows you to make every kind of healthy food for your whole family.
- This device is super easy to clean after using, and it saves a significant amount of time when making food.
- Plus, this machine is super beneficial when it comes to health because it can help you prevent several cardiovascular diseases. Because of the tiny amount of oil required to fry, the results will contain less than 80% of cholesterol than any

other normal fryer. The fan and grill allow air to circulate into the fryer and fry the food.

How an Air Fryer Works

- In an air fryer, there is a cooking chamber in which the actual cooking process takes place. Moreover, there is a drip tray placed into the air fryer basket, which allows you to cook crispy and tasty food.
- An automated temperature controller in the air fryer plays an important role in determining how the final product will come out.
- The digital screen and touchpad have made this device user-friendly because now users can control the device easily.
- The buzzer will automatically inform you when the food is done.

How to Start Cooking in an Air Fryer

To start cooking in an air fryer, you just need to spray the fryer basket with some cooking spray or put in a little cooking oil and adjust the temperature with time. Some recipes require shaking the basket halfway while cooking. In an air fryer, you can cook every kind of modern and traditional dish easily, including vegetables, patties, kebabs, chips, cakes, pastries, skewers, vegan fajitas, curly fries, muffins, pizzas, quiches, cupcakes, toasts, macaroni, and many more, without creating any kind of mess. This equipment is highly suitable for those who want to make food in an easier and healthier way.

How to Clean and Maintain Your Air Fryer

- You can easily wash your air fryer basket, pan, and, the tray after use with the help of hot water and any dishwashing soap.

- Dry out the parts completely with a clean cloth after washing before placing them back into air fryer.

- To remove any remaining food from the air fryer pan or basket, use a sponge.

- Always place the air fryer away from a wall or any other machinery while cooking. Make sure you use a clean air fryer every time you cook.

- Every food needs a different time and temperature to cook. Adjust the temperature and time according to the food or recipe and make sure that the food is not overcooked.

- After using your air fryer, clean it from the inside and outside.

- When done cooking, always make sure that the air fryer is no longer connected.

- Try to use light-colored pans for your air fryer. Otherwise, it will absorb more heat, and the food at the bottom will remain uncooked.

Cooking Conversion Charts

Weight Conversion	
15g	½ oz
30g	1 oz
60g	2 oz
85g	3 oz
110g	4 oz
140g	5 oz
170g	6 oz
200g	7 oz
225g	8 oz
255g	9 oz
280g	10 oz
310g	11 oz
340g	12 oz
370g	13 oz
400g	14 oz
425g	15 oz
450g	1 lb.

Liquid Volume Measurements

Tablespoons	Teaspoons	Fluid Ounces	Cups
16	48	8 fl. oz	1
12	36	6 fl. oz	¾
8	24	4 fl. oz	½
5 ½	16	2 ⅔ fl. oz	⅓
4	12	2 fl. oz	¼
1	3	0.5 fl. oz	1/16

Liquid Volume Conversion

Cups / Tablespoons	Fl. Ounces	Milliliters
1 cup	8 fl. oz	240 ml
¾ cup	6 fl. oz	180 ml
⅔ cup	5 fl. oz	150 ml
½ cup	4 fl. oz	120 ml
⅓ cup	2 ½ fl. oz	75 ml
¼ cup	2 fl. oz	60 ml
⅛ cup	1 fl. oz	30 ml
1 tablespoon	½ fl. oz	15 ml

Teaspoon / Tablespoon	Milliliters
1 tsp	5ml
2 tsp	10ml
1 Tbsp	15ml
2 Tbsp	30ml
3 Tbsp	45ml

Teaspoon / Tablespoon	Milliliters
4 Tbsp	60ml
5 Tbsp	75ml
6 Tbsp	90ml
7 Tbsp	105ml

Temperature Conversions	
Celsius	Fahrenheit
54 °C	130 °F
60 °C	140 °F
65 °C	150 °F
71 °C	160 °F
76 °C	170 °F
82 °C	180 °F
87 °C	190 °F
93 °C	200 °F
100 °C	212 °F
120 °C	250 °F
150 °C	300 °F
160 °C	320 °F
180 °C	360 °F
190 °C	380 °F
200 °C	400 °F
220 °C	425 °F

Mashed Potato Cakes

Make these cinnamon flavored mashed potato cakes for your breakfast and top them with tomato sauce and some vegan cheese. Your kids will love these cakes.

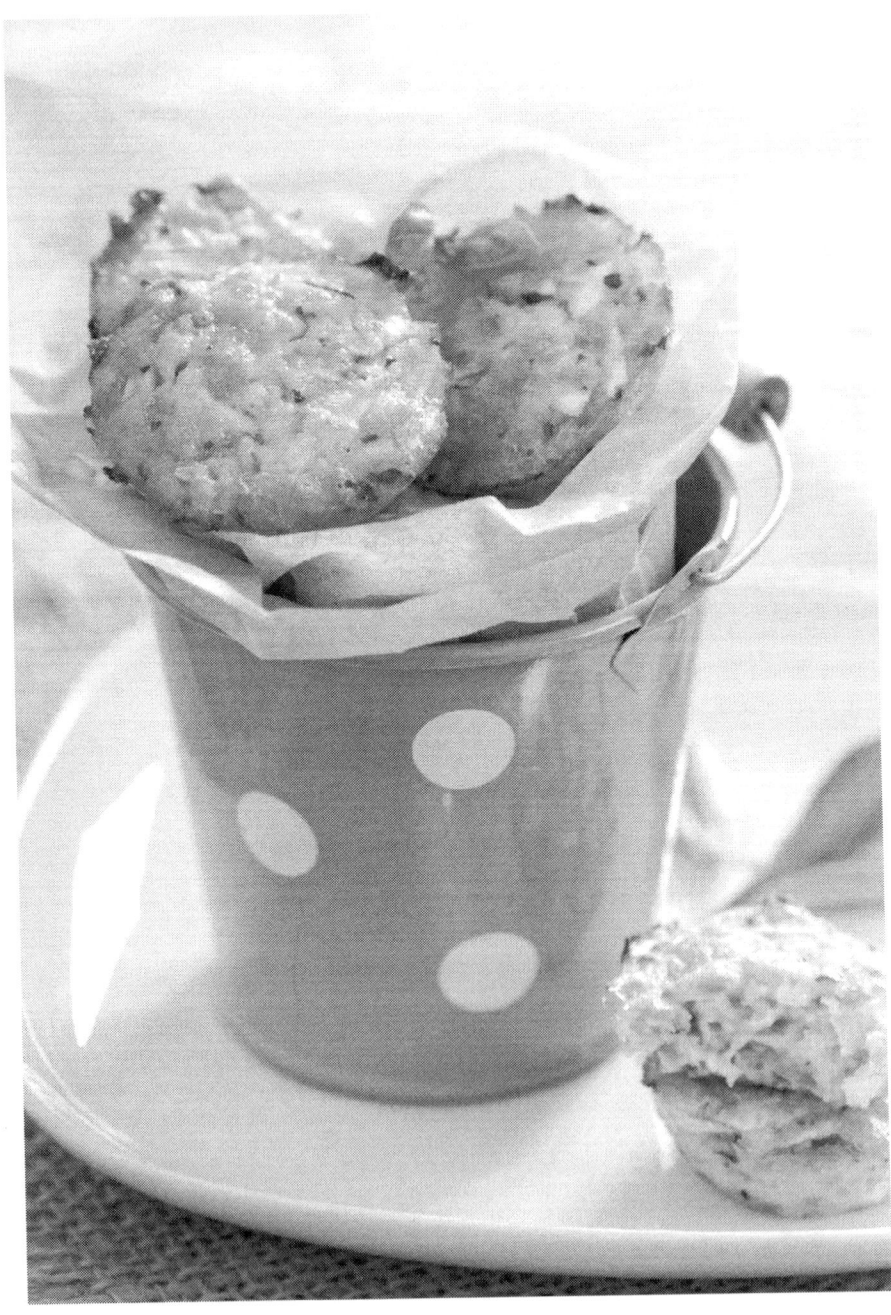

Serving: 4

Prep Time: 5 minutes

Cook Time: 8 minutes

Ingredients

- 4 large potatoes, boiled, peeled
- 1 bread slice
- 2 tablespoon cilantro, chopped
- 1 medium onion, chopped
- ¼ teaspoon cinnamon powder
- ¼ teaspoon cumin powder / chili
- ¼ teaspoon oregano
- ¼ teaspoon salt
- ¼ teaspoon black pepper
- 1 pinch salt

How To

1. In a food processor add potatoes, cinnamon powder, cilantro, cumin powder, oregano, onion, bread slice, salt, and black pepper, the process for 1 minute.
2. Transfer 3-4 tablespoons of mixture into greased muffin tins and press a little.
3. Preheat your Air Fryer to a temperature of 400°F (200°C).
4. Place muffin tins into air fryer basket and cook for 8 minutes.
5. Serve!

Nutrition Facts (Per Serving)

- Energy (calories): 170 kcal
- Protein: 3.67 g
- Fat: 0.4 g
- Carbohydrates: 38.83 g
- Dietary Fiber: 3.8

Air Fried Spicy Potatoes

These spicy potatoes are going to be the perfect meal for your lunch. Make this simple but delicious potato delight and serve with rice or yogurt sauce.

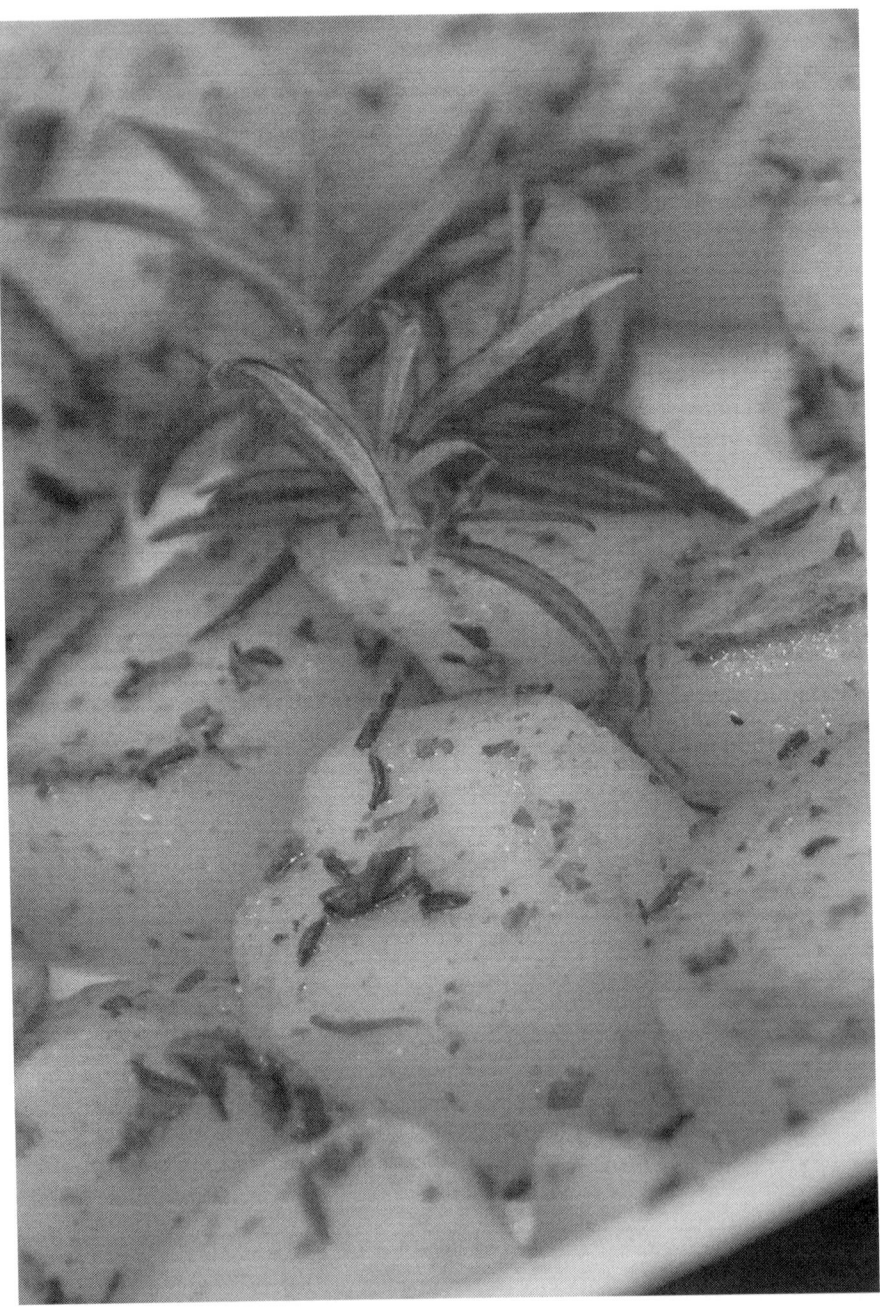

Serving: 4

Prep Time: 3 minutes

Cook Time: 12 minutes

Ingredients

- 1-pound potatoes, diced
- 1 teaspoon black pepper
- ¼ teaspoon nutmeg powder
- 1 teaspoon salt
- 1 tablespoons all-purpose flour
- ½ teaspoon cinnamon powder
- ½ teaspoon cumin powder
- 2 tablespoons olive oil
- 1 teaspoon basil leaves, chopped

How To

1. Pre-heat your Air Fryer to a temperature of 400°F (200°C).
2. In a bowl add potatoes, olive oil, flour, salt, black pepper, nutmeg powder, cumin powder, and cinnamon powder, mix well.
3. Now transfer potatoes in fryer basket and cook for 12 minutes.
4. Shake fryer basket after every 3 minutes.
5. When done put serving dish and top with basil leaves.
6. Serve!

Nutrition Facts (Per Serving)

- Energy (calories): 160 kcal
- Fat: 1g
- Dietary Fiber: 0g
- Protein: 25g
- Carbohydrates: 10g

Appealing Potato Kebabs

If you are craving for a quick and delicious lunch, then must try out this one. These potato kebabs are crunchy from outside and soft from inside. Serve them with any sauce or ketchup and enjoy.

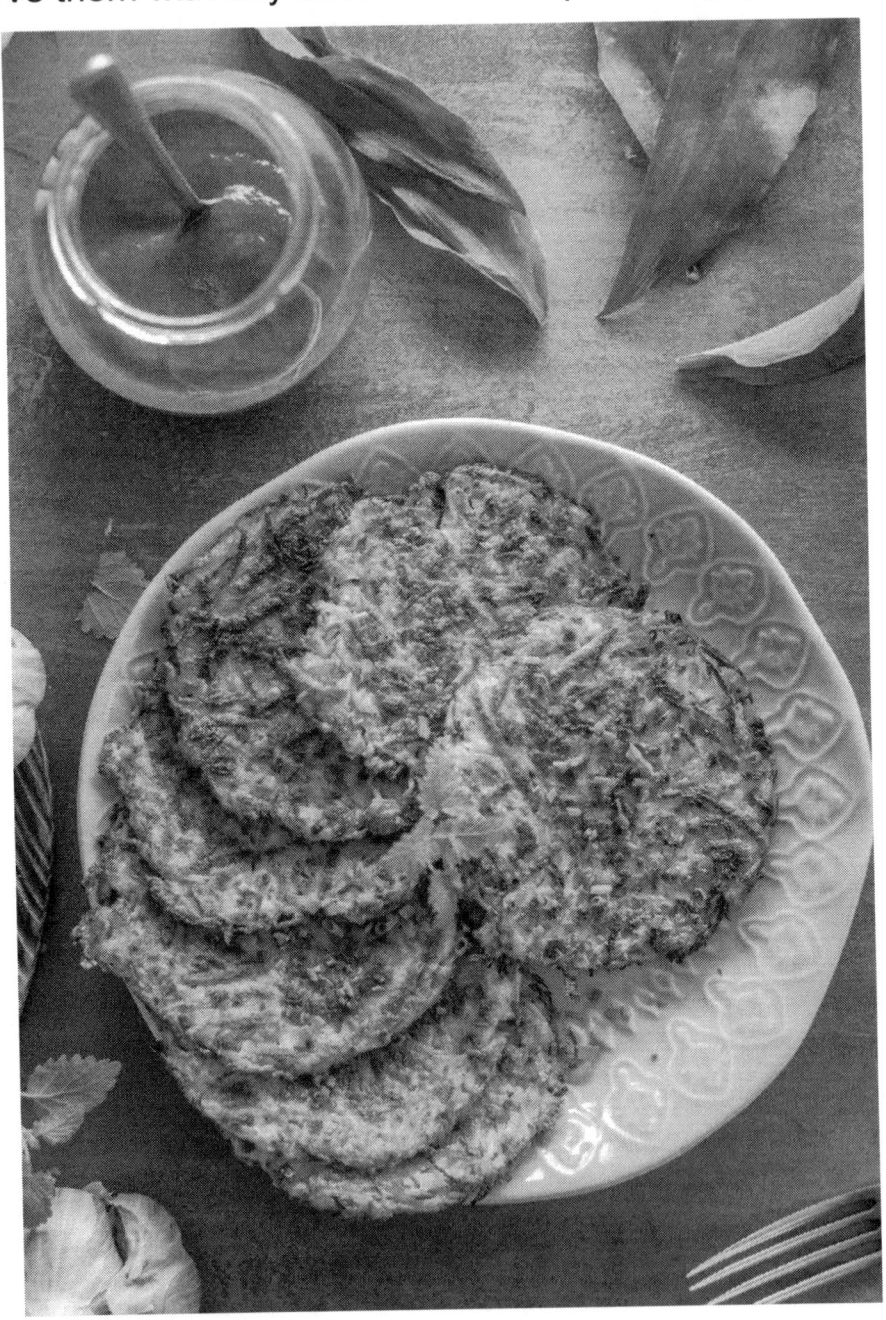

Serving: 4

Prep Time: 10 minutes

Cook Time: 10 minutes

Ingredients

- 5 potatoes, boiled, peeled
- 2 bread slices
- 1 onion, chopped
- 2 tablespoons coriander leaves, chopped
- ¼ teaspoon cinnamon powder
- ¼ teaspoon chili powder
- ¼ teaspoon salt
- ¼ teaspoon black pepper
- 2 tablespoons spring onion, chopped

How To

1. In a blender or food processor add potatoes, onion, spring onion, salt, chili powder, cinnamon powder, black pepper, and coriander, blend until combined well.
2. Preheat Air Fryer at the temperature of 400°F (200°C).
3. Make round kebabs with the mixture and place them in air fryer basket.
4. Cook for 5 minutes then flip the sides and cook again for another 5 minutes.

Nutrition Facts (Per Serving)

- Energy (calories): 180 kcal
- Fat: 0.5g
- Dietary Fiber: 4.2 g
- Protein: 4.48g
- Carbohydrates: 42g

Whole Baked Cauliflower

This whole cauliflower is super tasty to try. Sprinkle all spices on cauliflower and bake it in your Air Fryer at the temperature of 400°F. Serve it with roasted bell pepper and chili sauce.

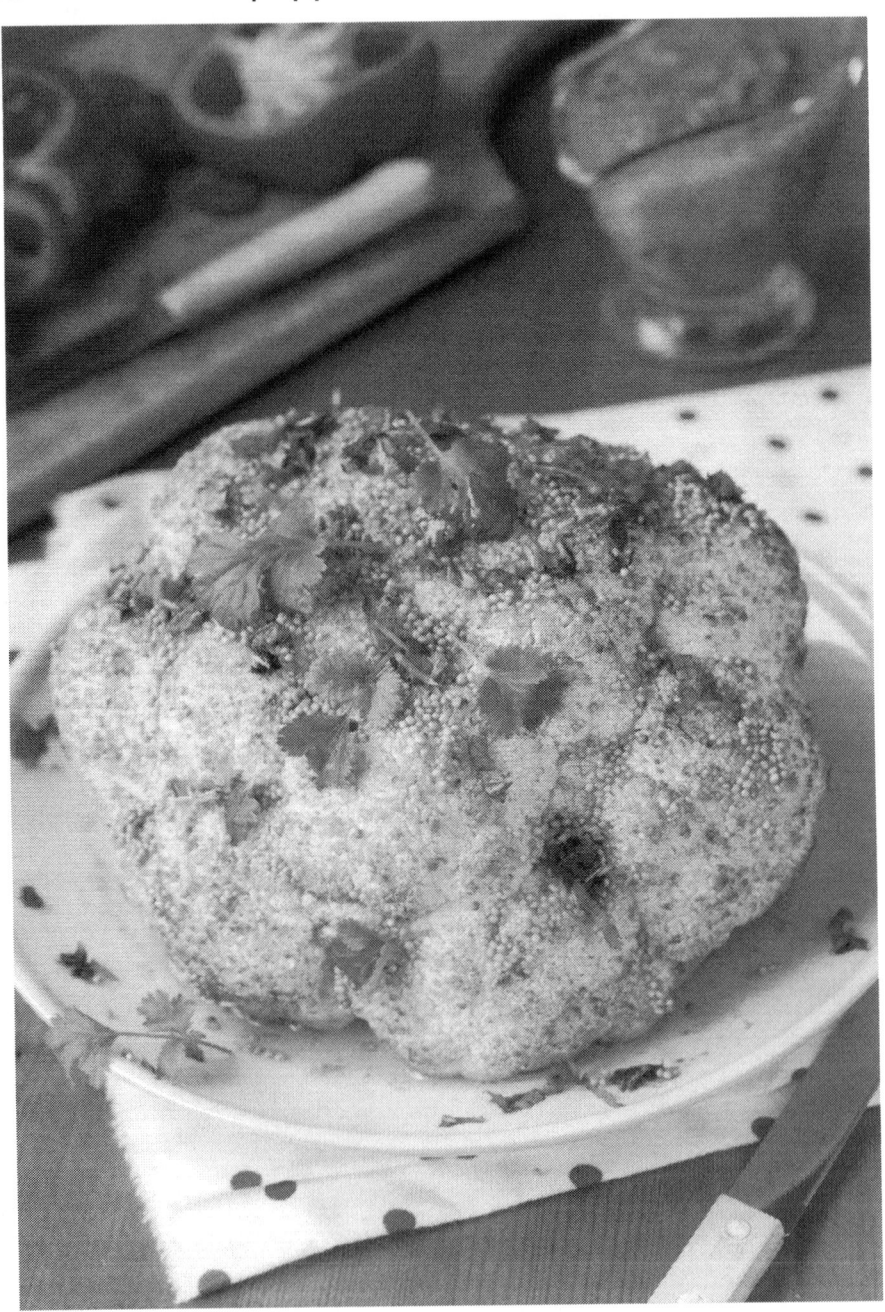

Serving: 2

Prep Time: 1 minute

Cook Time: 12 minutes

Ingredients

- 1 whole cauliflower
- 1 tablespoon ginger powder
- 1 teaspoon garlic powder
- ½ teaspoon salt
- ¼ teaspoon white pepper
- 2 tablespoons olive oil

How To

1. Preheat your Air Fryer to a temperature of 400°F (200°C).
2. Brush cauliflower with olive oil.
3. Sprinkle it with salt, pepper, garlic powder and ginger powder.
4. Transfer it to air fryer basket and leave to cook for 12 minutes.
5. Serve and enjoy.

Nutrition Facts (Per Serving)

- Energy (calories): 209 kcal
- Fat: 9g
- Dietary Fiber: 0g
- Protein: 15g
- Carbohydrates: 20g

Balsamic Cabbage Steaks

This unique and flavorful cabbage delight is packed with bursting flavors. Just sprinkle salt, thyme, black pepper and drizzle balsamic vinegar and some olive oil. Cook in air fryer for just 4 minutes and enjoy.

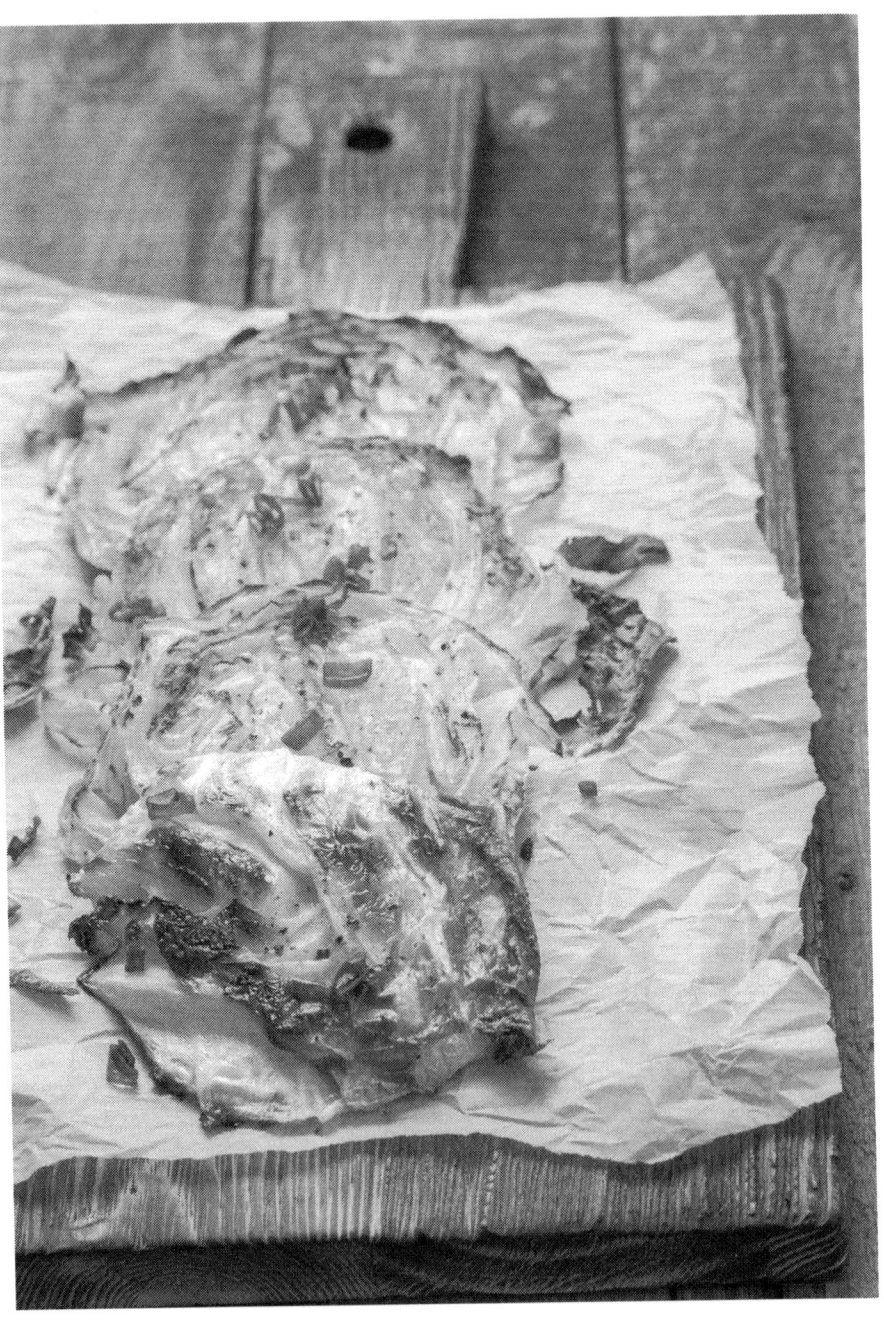

Serving: 2

Prep Time: 1 minute

Cook Time: 4 minutes

Ingredients

- 1 whole cabbages, cut into slices
- ½ teaspoon black pepper
- ¼ teaspoon salt
- ½ teaspoon thyme
- 2 tablespoons balsamic vinegar
- 1 teaspoon olive oil

How To

1. In a large bowl add black pepper, salt, thyme, vinegar, and olive oil, mix well.
2. Preheat your Air Fryer to a temperature of 400°F (200°C).
3. Transfer cabbage slice into air fryer basket and brush them with balsamic sauce.
4. Place to cook for 4 minutes.
5. Serve!

Nutrition Facts (Per Serving)

- Energy (calories): 260 kcal
- Fat: 4g
- Dietary Fiber: 12g
- Protein: 8g
- Carbohydrates: 45g

Mouth-Melting Broccoli Bites

Broccoli bites are filling and yummy dinner if you want to switch from for normal food routine. Make these bites and serve them with any sauce or dip. You can also make these bites for your tea time party.

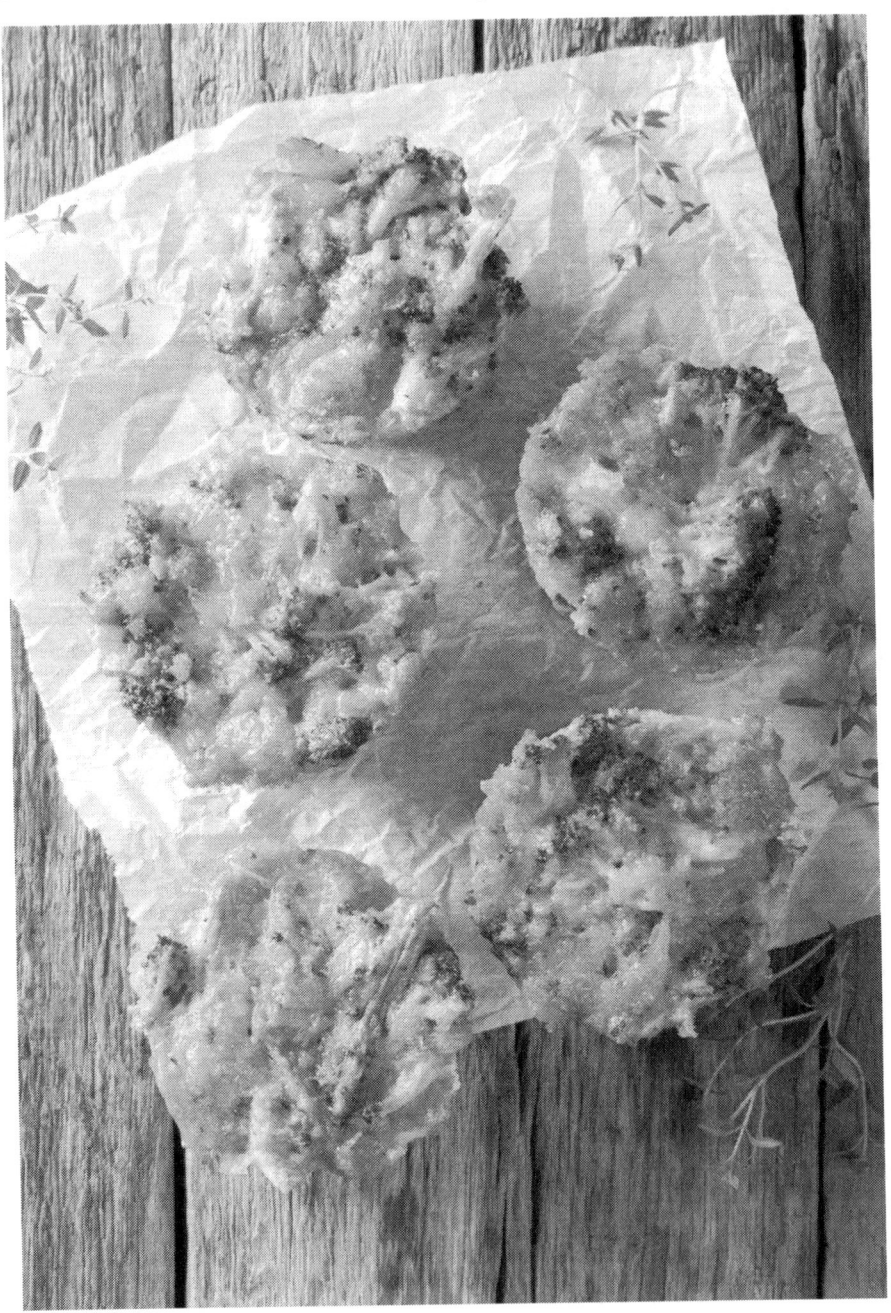

Serving: 4

Prep Time: 5 minutes

Cook Time: 8 minutes

Ingredients

- 1 ½ cup broccoli, boiled
- 1 cup gram flour
- 3 tablespoons corn flour
- ¼ teaspoon cinnamon powder
- ½ teaspoon dry coriander powder
- ¼ teaspoon nutmeg powder
- ½ teaspoon chili powder
- ¼ teaspoon salt
- ¼ cup water

How To

1. In a bowl add broccoli and mash it potato masher for 1-2 minutes.
2. Add gram flour, corn flour, cinnamon powder, nutmeg powder, salt, and chili powder, mix.
3. Add water gradually and make a thick batter.
4. Preheat Air Fryer at the temperature of 380°F (190°C).
5. Now take 1 tablespoon of batter into hand and shape it into round ball.
6. Transfer these balls to air fryer basket and cook for 4 minutes, then flip sides and cook again for 4 minutes.

Nutrition Facts (Per Serving)

- Energy (calories): 114 kcal
- Fat: 2g
- Dietary Fiber: 3.5g
- Protein: 6g
- Carbohydrates: 30g

Roasted Brussels Sprouts, Sweet Potatoes and Mushrooms

This simple option for your dinner is perfectly awesome. It's a unique combination of Brussels sprout, mushrooms and sweet potatoes in with some seasonings. You will enjoy your dinner.

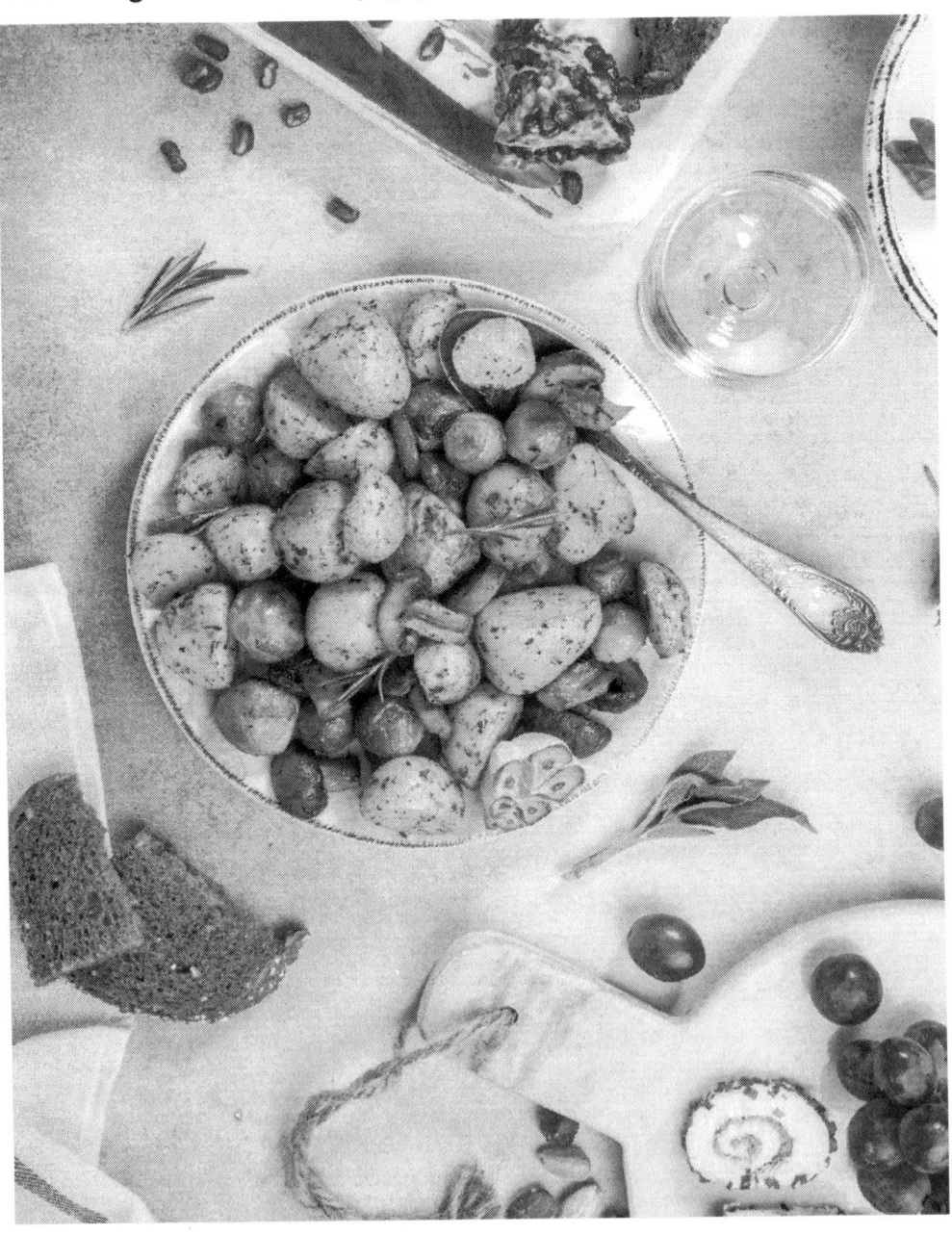

Serving: 2

Prep Time: 2 minutes

Cook Time: 8 minutes

Ingredients

- 1-pound brussels sprouts halved
- 1-pound sweet potatoes, peeled, cut into cubes
- ½ pound mushrooms halved
- Salt and black pepper, to taste
- 1 teaspoon olive oil
- 1 teaspoon soya sauce
- ½ teaspoon oregano
- ¼ teaspoon garlic powder

How To

1. Preheat Air Fryer at a temperature of 360°F (180°C).
2. Sprinkle salt, garlic powder, oregano, and pepper on brussels sprouts and sweet potatoes, drizzle olive oil and soya sauce toss to combine.
3. Transfer to fryer basket and leave to cook for 8 minutes.
4. Shake fryer basket after every 2 minutes.
5. Serve!

Nutrition Facts (Per Serving)

- Energy (calories): 225 kcal
- Protein: 13.78 g
- Fat: 4.18 g
- Carbohydrates: 43.18 g
- Dietary Fiber 21.3 g

Roasted Beetroots with Onion

Roasted beetroots give awesome flavors with onion. Here are golden and red beetroots, but you can add any kind according to your desire.

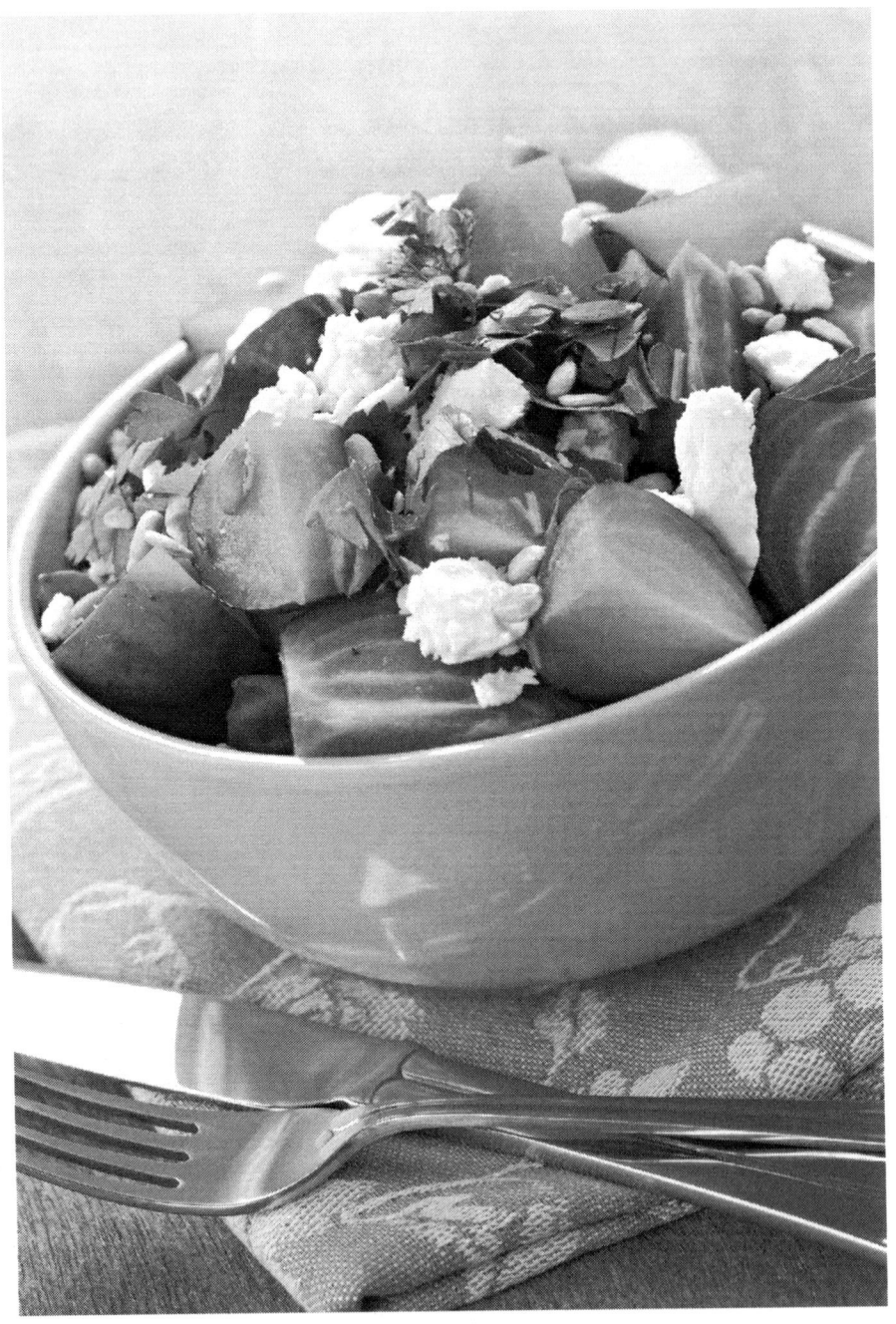

Serving: 4

Prep Time: 1 minute

Cook Time: 8 minutes

Ingredients

- 4 onions, peeled, halved
- 6 beetroots, peeled, halved
- 5 golden beetroots, peeled, halved
- ½ cup tofu
- 1 teaspoon mixed herbs
- 1 tablespoon coconut oil
- 1 tablespoon lime juice
- ¼ teaspoon salt
- ¼ teaspoon black pepper

How To

1. Preheat your Air Fryer to a temperature of 360°F (180°C).
2. Transfer onions and beetroots into air fryer basket.
3. Sprinkle salt and pepper, toss to combine.
4. Leave to prepare for 8 minutes.
5. Shake the basket of air fryer after every 2 minutes.
6. When done put into a bowl and drizzle coconut oil and lime juice.
7. Sprinkle mix herbs and stir well
8. Finally sprinkle with tofu.

Nutrition Facts (Per Serving)

- Energy (calories): 235 kcal
- Protein: 9.87 g
- Fat: 8.9 g
- Carbohydrates: 32.26 g
- Dietary Fiber 8.2 g

Turmeric Flavored Mashed Potato Stuffed Fritters

Mashed potato stuffed fritters are flavored with a traditional Indian spice that is famous as turmeric powder. These fritters are super tempting and quick.

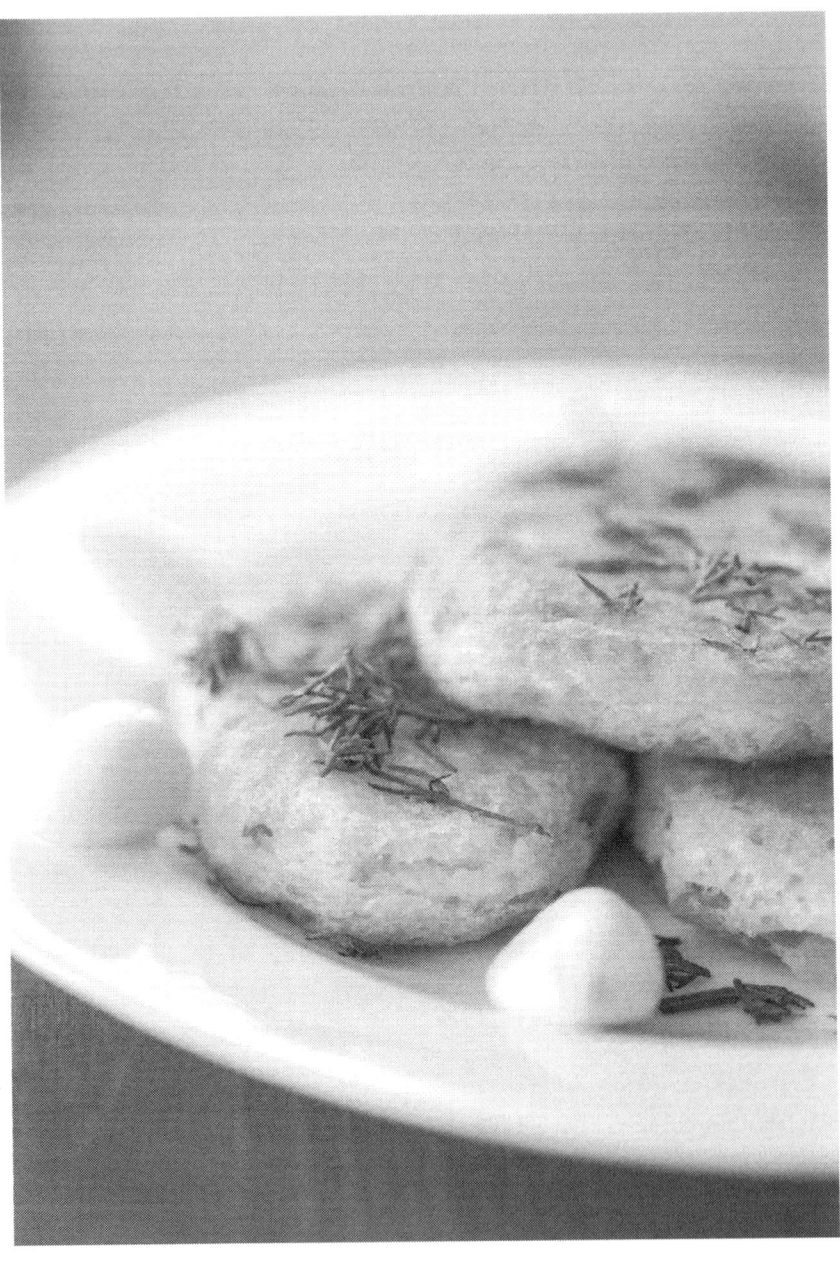

Serving: 12

Prep Time: 5 minutes

Cook Time: 8 minutes

Ingredients

- 1 cup all-purpose flour
- ¼ cup water
- 4 potatoes, boiled, peeled
- 1 onion, chopped
- ¼ teaspoon turmeric powder
- ¼ teaspoon garlic powder
- ½ teaspoon black pepper
- ¼ teaspoon salt
- ¼ teaspoon cumin seeds
- 2 tablespoons cilantro, chopped

How To

1. Preheat Air Fryer to a temperature of 380°F (190°C).
2. Take a bowl and add in flour and water, mix well and make a thick paste.
3. Mash potatoes with a potato masher and add salt, pepper, cilantro, turmeric powder, onion, garlic powder, and cumin seeds, mix well.
4. Now make fritters with potato mixture and dip each into flour paste.
5. Transfer them to air fryer basket, leave to cook for 8 minutes.
6. Serve!

Nutrition Facts (Per Serving)

- Energy (calories): 82 kcal
- Protein: 2.06 g
- Fat: 0.17 g
- Carbohydrates: 18.06 g
- Dietary Fiber 1.3 g

Crispy Onion Pakoras

These crispy and spicy onion pakoras are traditional Indian appetizer. These are made up of onion slices, gram flour, green chilies, mint, cilantro, and few spices.

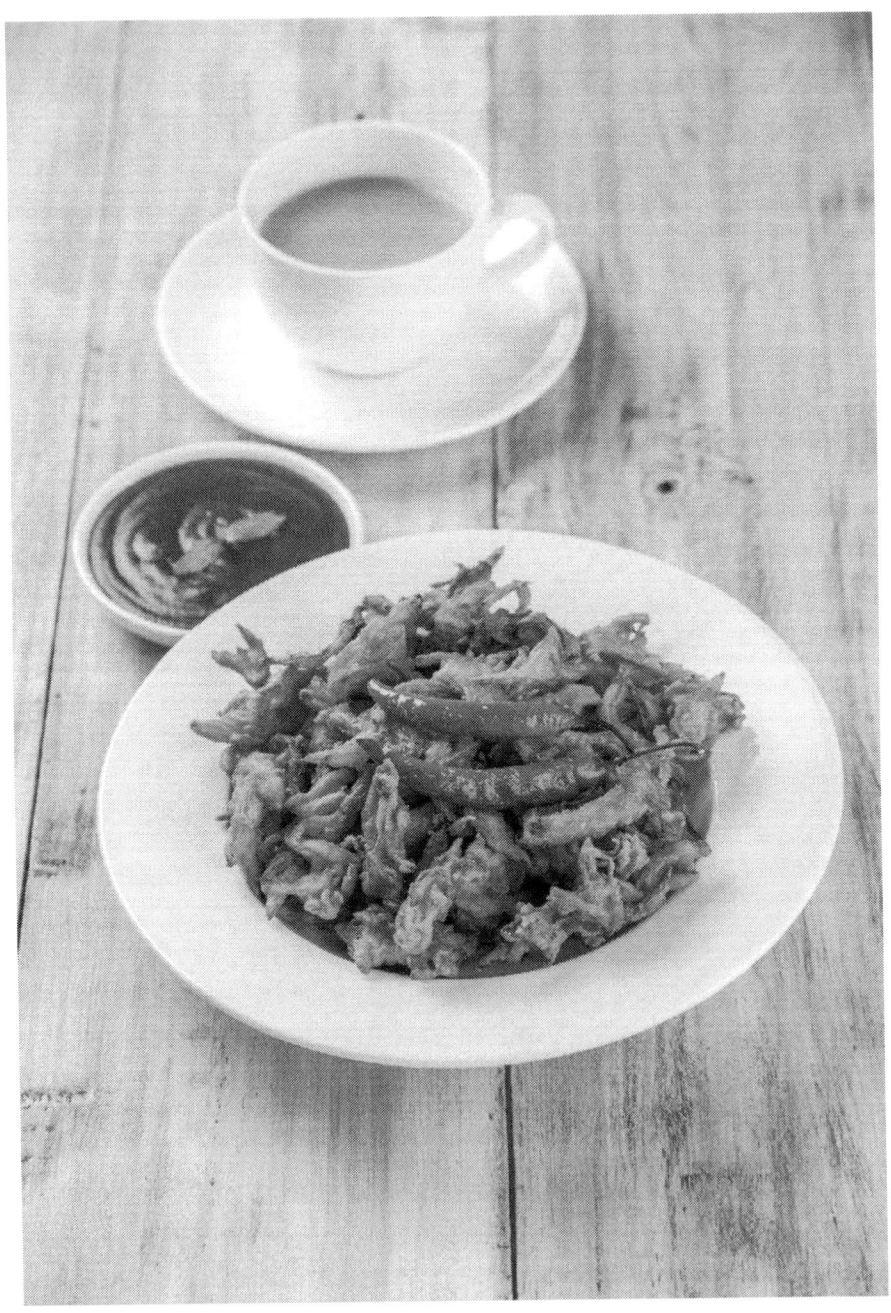

Serving: 8

Prep Time: 5 minutes

Cook Time: 4 minutes

Ingredients

- 3 onions thinly sliced
- 1 cup gram flour
- 1 teaspoon salt
- ¼ teaspoon chili powder
- ¼ teaspoon cumin powder
- ¼ teaspoon cinnamon powder
- ¼ teaspoon dry coriander powder
- 2 tablespoons cilantro, chopped
- 2 tablespoons mint leaves, chopped
- 2 green chilies, chopped
- ¼ cup water

How To

1. Preheat Air Fryer at a temperature of 360°F (180°C).
2. In a large bowl add onion, flour, salt, chili powder, coriander leaves, mint, green chilies, cumin powder, cinnamon powder, and dry coriander powder, mix well.
3. Now add water gradually to make a thick batter.
4. Place 1-2 tablespoons of mixture into air fryer basket at 1 inch apart from each fritter and leave to cook for 4 minutes.
5. Serve with chili sauce!

Nutrition Facts (Per Serving)

- Energy (calories): 62 kcal
- Protein: 3.06 g
- Fat: 0.84 g
- Carbohydrates: 10.65 g
- Dietary Fiber 2 g

Spring Onion and Cabbage Filled Wontons

These wontons are super yummy and can be served with garlic sauce or tomato sauce. Bake them in your air fryer for just 8 minutes and enjoy their magic.

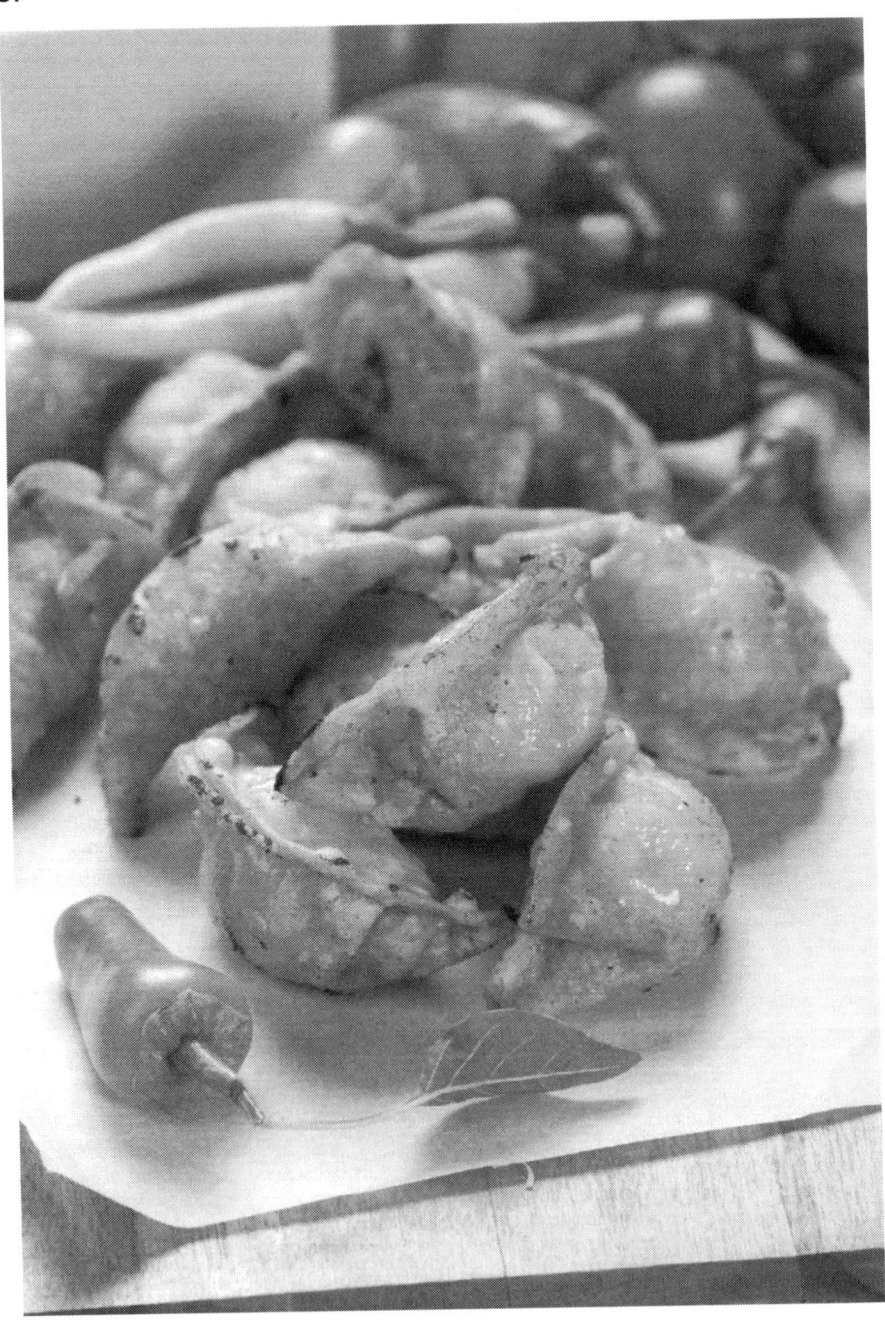

Serving: 8

Prep Time: 5 minutes

Cook Time: 8 minutes

Ingredients

- 8 wonton sheets
- 1 cup spring onion, chopped
- 1 cup cabbage, shredded
- 1 teaspoon salt
- ½ teaspoon black pepper
- 1 tablespoon lime juice

How To

1. In a bowl add cabbages, onion, salt, and black pepper, mix well.
2. Place 1-2 tablespoons of mixture on each wonton sheet and brush its edges with water.
3. Take one edge of each wonton and flip it over filling.
4. Make patterns with folk on edges.
5. Make all wontons in the same way.
6. Preheat your Air Fryer to a temperature of 360°F (180°C).
7. Place wontons into air fryer basket and leave to prepare for 8 minutes.
8. Serve and enjoy.

Nutrition Facts (Per Serving)

- Calories: 304 kcal
- Fat: 5g
- Dietary Fiber: 0g
- Protein: 20g
- Carbohydrates: 42g

Crispy Masala Tofu

These crispy tofu's are worth to try; you will forget to try any other dish after eating this one. It's not only simple to make but packed with enchanting flavors.

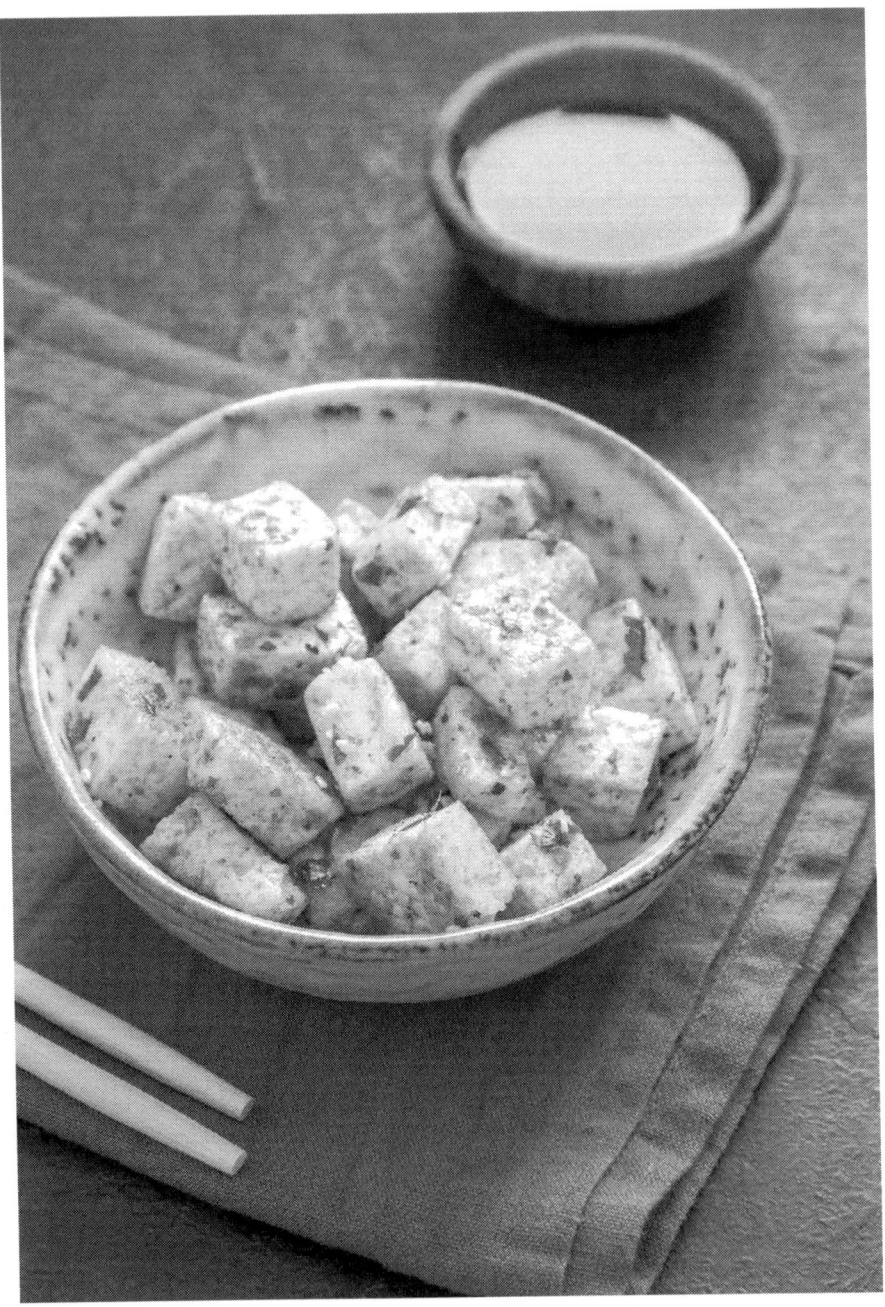

Serving: 4

Prep Time: 2 minutes

Cook Time: 8 minutes

Ingredients

- 1-pound tofu
- ¼ teaspoon black pepper
- ¼ teaspoon salt
- 4 tablespoons rice flour
- 1 tablespoon olive oil
- 2 tablespoons parsley
- ¼ cup spring onions, chopped

How To

1. Preheat Air Fryer to a temperature of 360°F (180°C).
2. Drizzle olive oil on tofu and toss.
3. Sprinkle salt, pepper, and rice flour on tofu and mix well until coated.
4. Put to fryer basket and leave to cook for 8 minutes.
5. Shake air fryer basket after 2 minutes.
6. Transfer to serving dish and top with parsley and spring onion.
7. Serve and enjoy!

Nutrition Facts (Per Serving)

- Energy (calories): 155 kcal
- Protein: 10.07 g
- Fat: 9.1 g
- Carbohydrates: 10.38 g
- Dietary Fiber 1.3 g

Rosemary Zest Roasted Potatoes

These roasted potatoes are extremely mouth melting. You will not resist to make them again; it's a bet! It's a quick dish which can be done in few minutes or anytime.

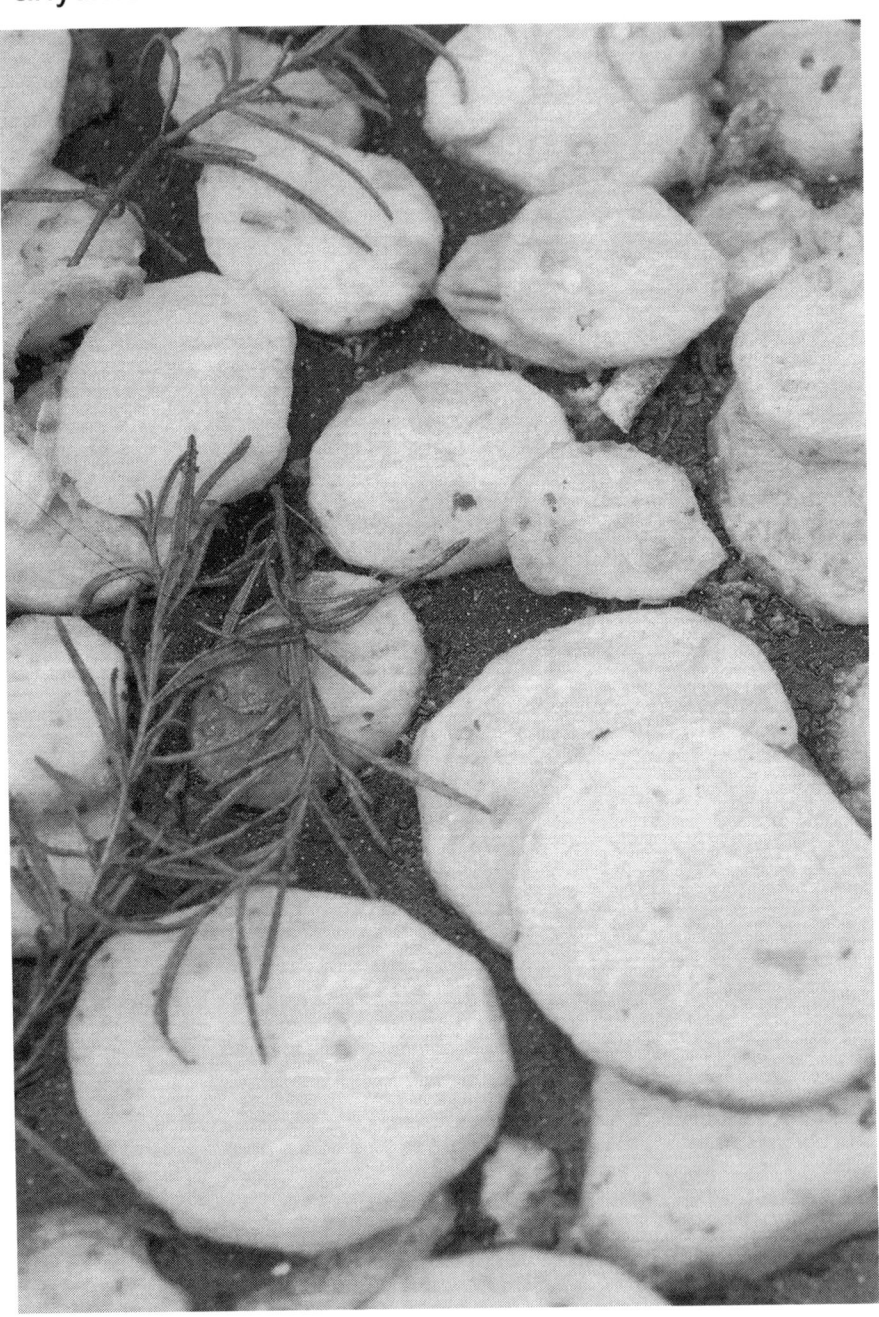

Serving: 4

Prep Time: 1 minute

Cook Time: 8 minutes

Ingredients

- 5 medium potatoes, slices
- ¼ teaspoon salt
- ¼ teaspoon black pepper
- 1 tablespoon rosemary
- ¼ teaspoon cinnamon powder
- 1 teaspoon olive oil

How To

1. Preheat Air Fryer to a temperature of 360°F (180°C).
2. Transfer potatoes in air fryer and drizzle olive oil, toss to combine and leave to cook for 8 minutes.
3. Shake air fryer basket after every 2 minutes.
4. When done transfer into bowl and season with cinnamon powder, salt, black pepper, and rosemary.
5. Serve!

Nutrition Facts (Per Serving)

- Energy (calories): 216 kcal
- Protein: 5.42 g
- Fat: 1.4 g
- Carbohydrates: 46.85 g
- Dietary Fiber 6,1 g

Bottle Gourd and Split Gram Patties

These patties are made up boiled bottle gourd, boiled split gram, mint leaves, gram flour, salt, chili flakes, and cumin powder. Its delicious dish for your table that everyone wants to enjoy.

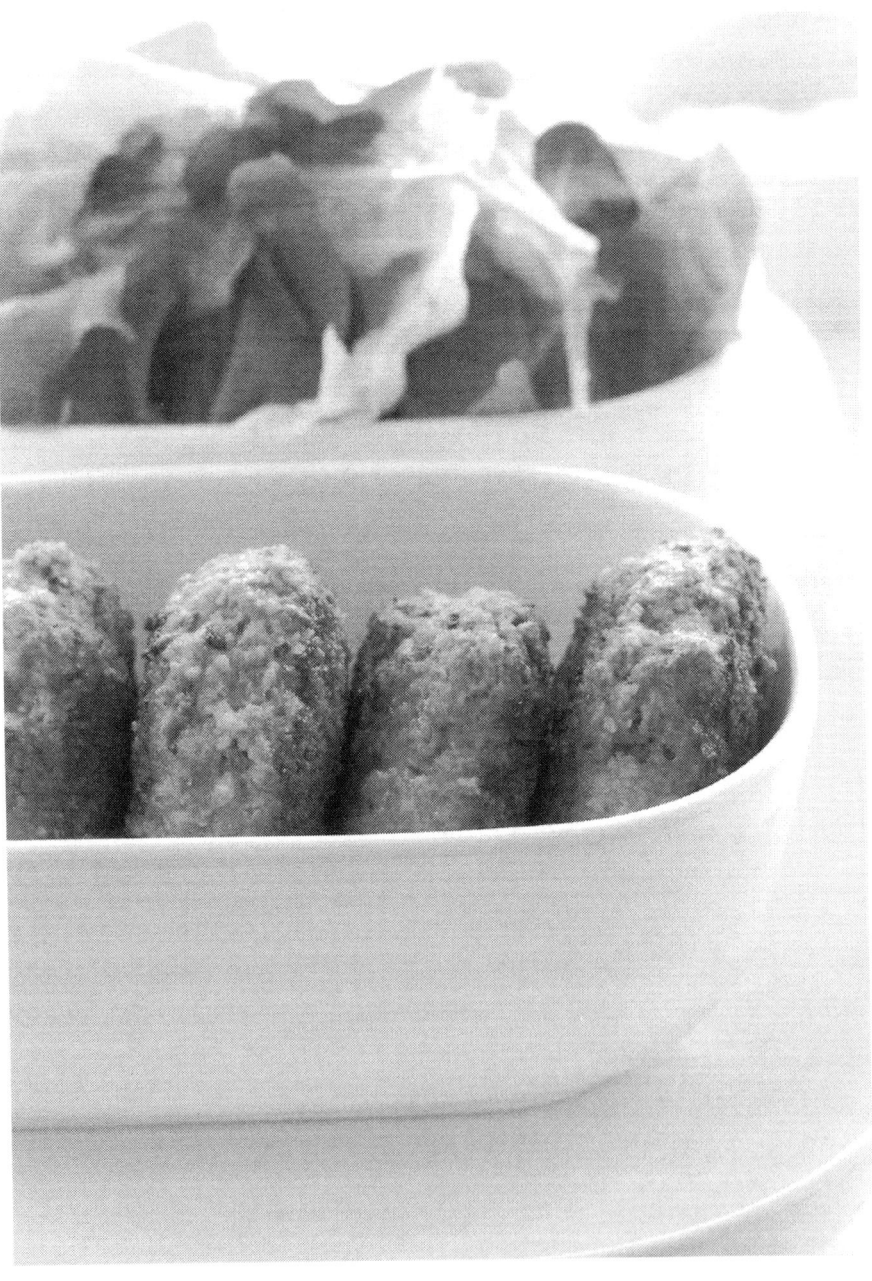

Serving: 8

Prep Time: 15 minutes

Cook Time: 8 minutes

Ingredients

- 1 cup bottle gourd, slices, boiled
- 1 cup split gram, boiled
- 1 bunch mint leaves
- ¼ teaspoon chili flakes
- ½ cup gram flour
- 1 tablespoon lime juice
- ¼ teaspoon salt
- ¼ teaspoon cumin powder
- 1 teaspoon olive oil

How To

1. Preheat your Air Fryer to a temperature of 360°F (180°C).
2. In a food processor add bottle gourd, split gram, mint leaves, gram flour, salt, chili flakes, cumin powder, olive oil, and lime juice, blend well.
3. Now make round and flatten patties with the mixture and place them into air fryer basket.
4. Leave to cook for 8 minutes.
5. Serve with chili sauce.

Nutrition Facts (Per Serving)

- Energy (calories): 49 kcal
- Protein: 2.12 g
- Fat: 1.1 g
- Carbohydrates: 8.16 g
- Dietary Fiber 1.9 g

Sweet Potato Garlic Chips

These garlic flavors sweet potatoes chips are perfect for everyone. Even your kids will enjoy a lot. You can also make these chips for your kid's lunch box.

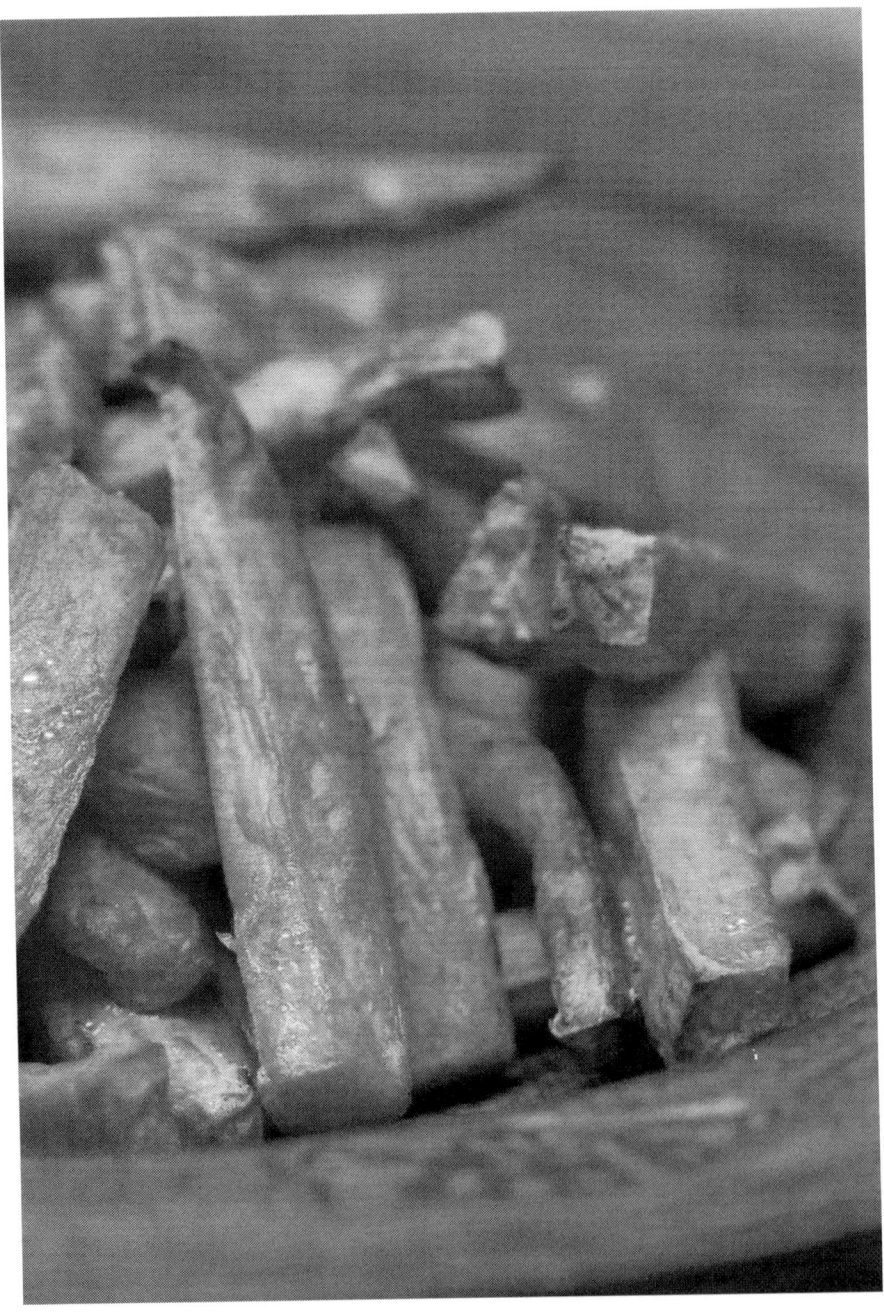

Serving: 4

Prep Time: 1 minute

Cook Time: 8 minutes

Ingredients

- 4 sweet potatoes, peeled, sliced
- ¼ teaspoon garlic powder
- ¼ teaspoon salt
- 1 teaspoon olive oil
- 1 teaspoon parsley, chopped

How To

1. Preheat Air Fryer at the temperature of 320°F (160°C).
2. Transfer chips into air fryer basket and drizzle olive oil.
3. Sprinkle salt and garlic powder, toss to combine.
4. Leave to cook for 8 minutes.
5. Shake air fryer basket after 2 minutes.
6. When done put on a serving platter and sprinkle parsley on top.

Nutrition Facts (Per Serving)

- Energy (calories): 123 kcal
- Protein: 2.08 g
- Fat: 1.19 g
- Carbohydrates: 26.32 g
- Dietary Fiber 3.9 g

Soya Sauce and Pepper Flavored Cauliflower

This giant cauliflower is super delicious that is made up simply with soya sauce and black pepper seasoning. Make it and serve hot with yogurt dip.

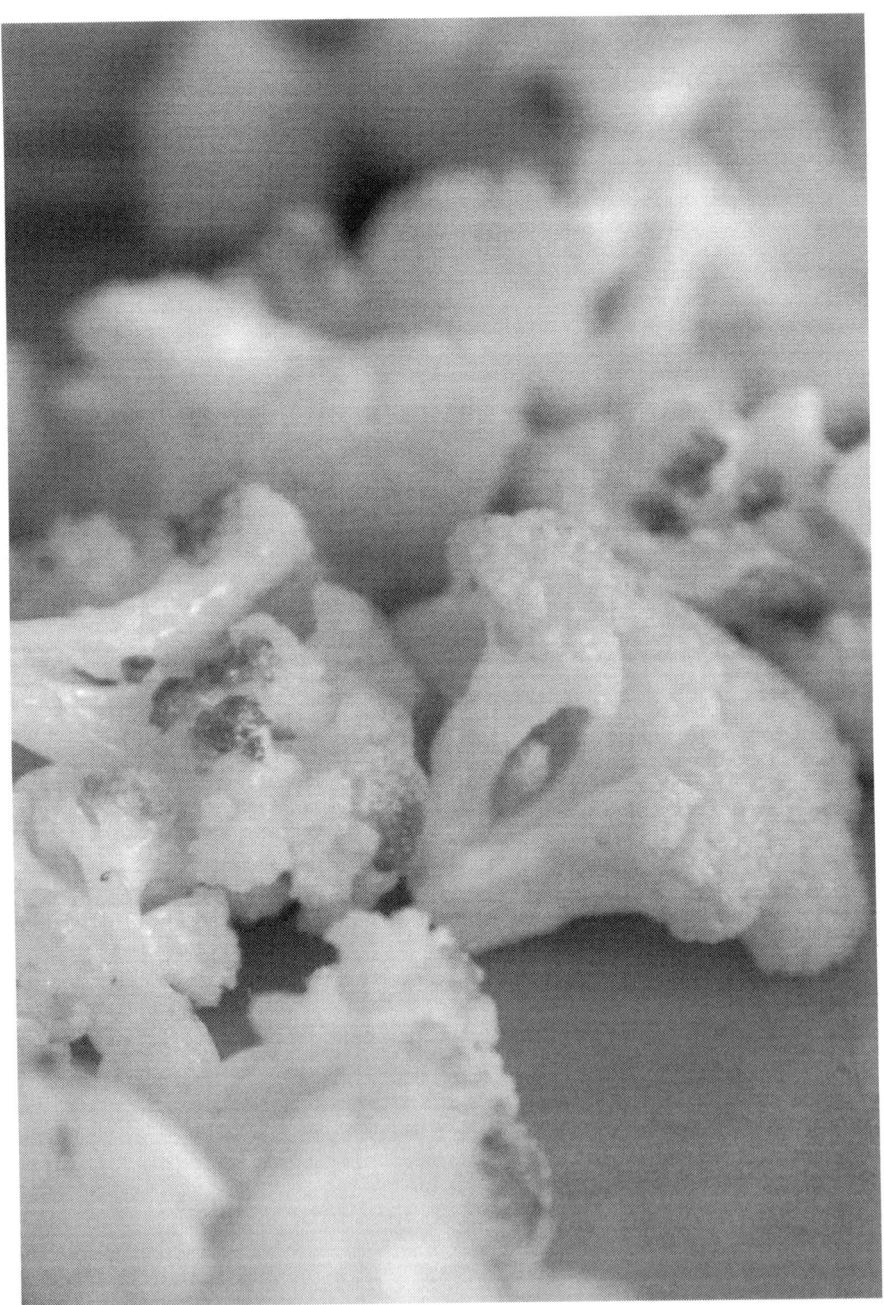

Serving: 2

Prep Time: 1 minute

Cook Time: 8 minutes

Ingredients

- 1 cauliflower, florets
- 3 tablespoons soya sauce
- 1 teaspoon black pepper
- ¼ teaspoon salt

How To

1. Preheat your Air Fryer to a temperature of 360°F (180°C).
2. In a bowl add soya sauce, salt, and pepper, mix well.
3. Brush cauliflower with soya sauce mixture and put it in air fryer basket.
4. Let to cook for 8 minutes.
5. Serve with yogurt.

Nutrition Facts (Per Serving)

- Energy (calories): 78 kcal
- Protein: 6.92 g
- Fat: 0.74 g
- Carbohydrates: 15.87 g
- Dietary Fiber 7.7 g

Turmeric Zest Potato and Cauliflower

This simple and light dish is packed with turmeric flavor. You will love to enjoy this dish with your friend and family.

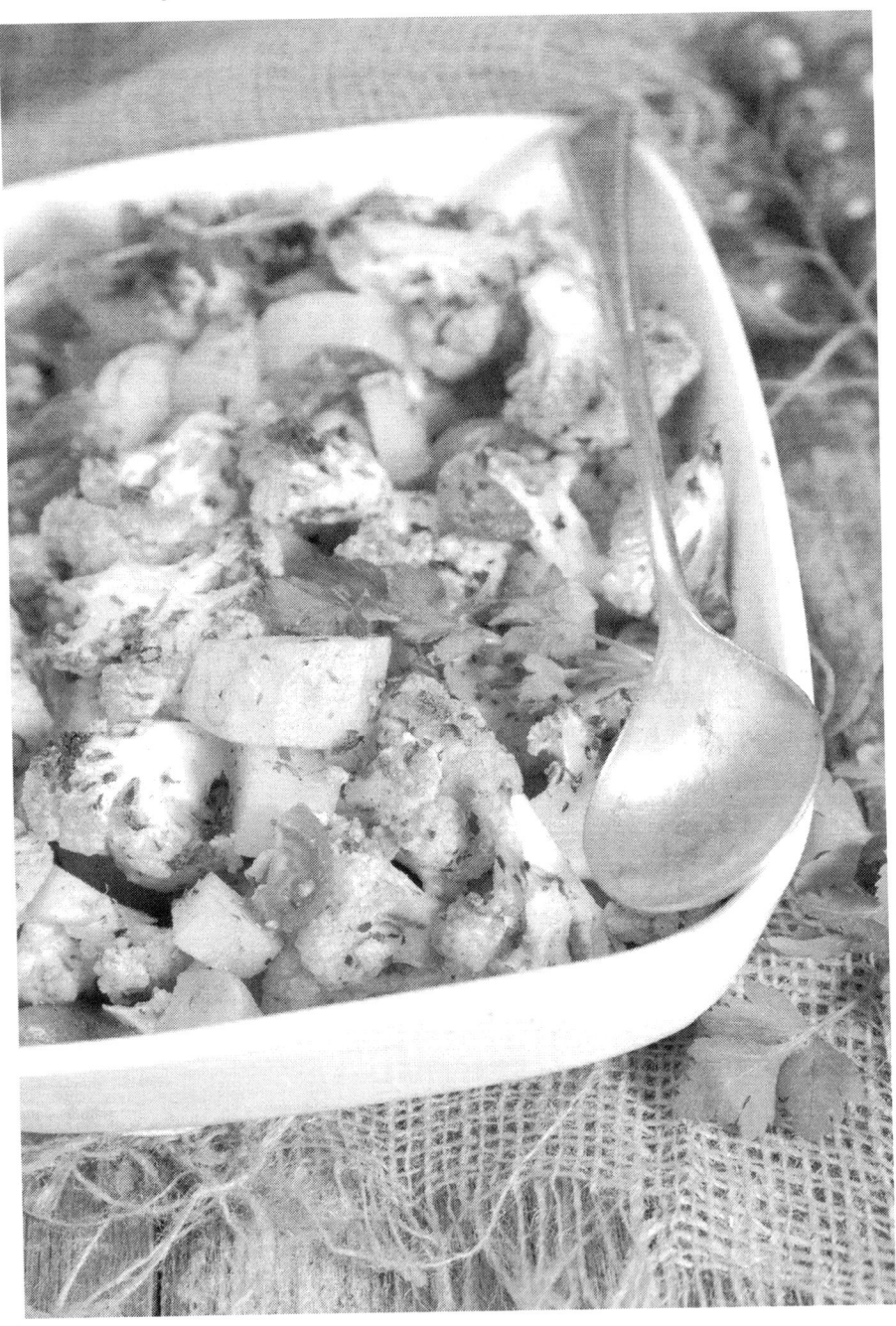

Serving: 4

Prep Time: 5 minutes

Cook Time: 12 minutes

Ingredients

- 2 cups cauliflower, florets
- 4 potatoes, peeled, diced
- ¼ teaspoon salt
- ¼ teaspoon turmeric powder
- ¼ teaspoon lime juice
- ¼ teaspoon vinegar
- 4 cherry tomatoes for serving

How To

1. In a large bowl add potatoes, cauliflower, salt, turmeric powder, vinegar, and lime juice, toss well to combine.
2. Preheat Air Fryer at the temperature of 380°F (190°C).
3. Put cauliflower and potatoes into air fryer basket and cook for 12 minutes.
4. Keep shaking the air fryer basket after every 2 minutes.
5. Serve with cherry tomatoes.

Nutrition Facts (Per Serving)

- Energy (calories): 178 kcal
- Protein: 5.35 g
- Fat: 0.35 g
- Carbohydrates: 40.03 g
- Dietary Fiber 5.8 g

Coriander and Chili Bites

Here is a unique and flavorful delight for you. This puffy coriander and chili bites are smooth and softened from inside and crunch from outside.

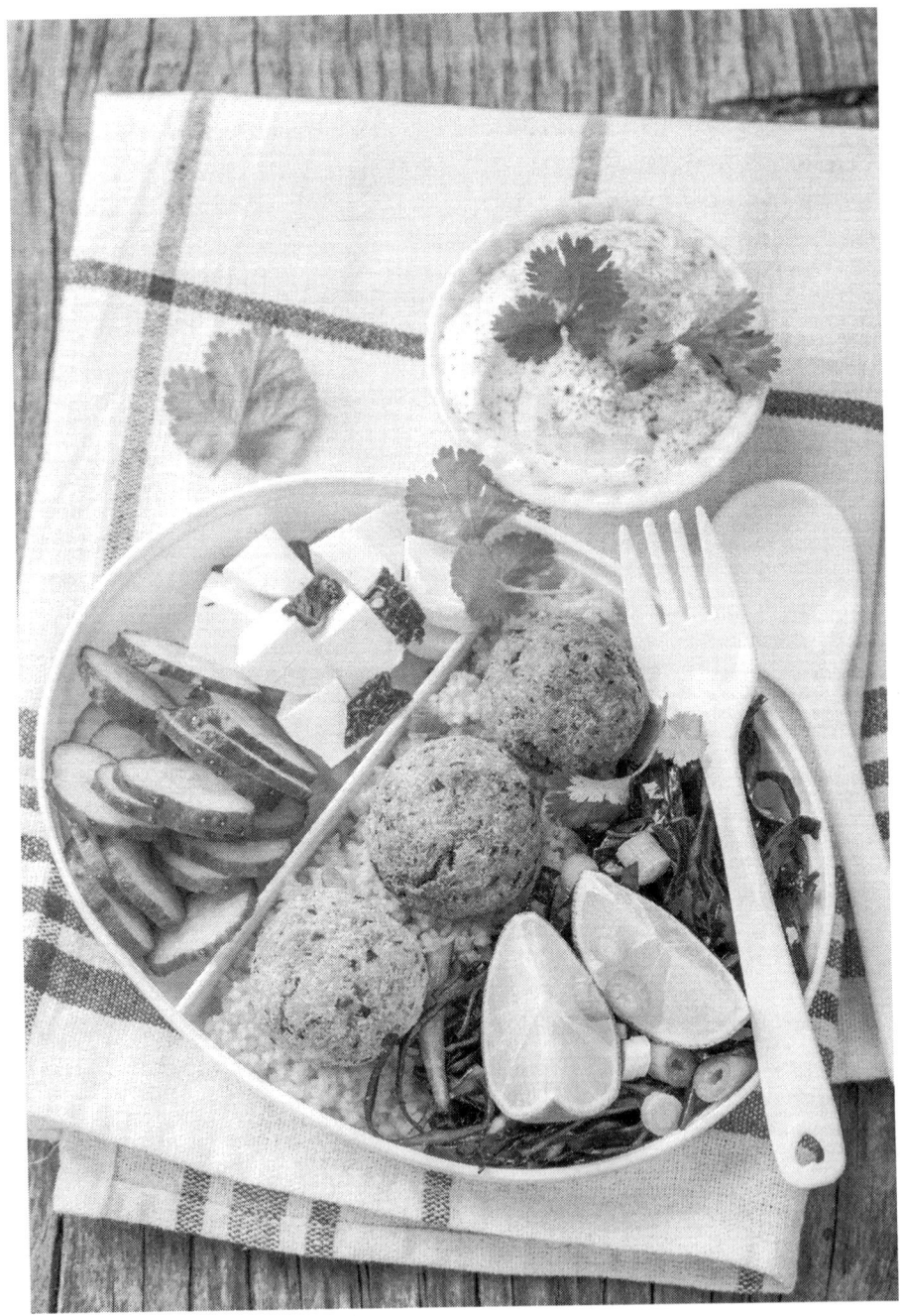

Serving: 6

Prep Time: 5 minutes

Cook Time: 8 minutes

Ingredients

- 1 cup gram flour
- ¼ cup corn flour
- ½ teaspoon black pepper
- ¼ teaspoon turmeric powder
- ¼ teaspoon cumin powder
- ¼ teaspoon cinnamon powder
- ¼ teaspoon dry coriander powder
- 1 bunch coriander leaves, chopped
- 3 green chilies, chopped
- 1 large pinch baking soda

How To

1. Preheat your Air Fryer to a temperature of 380°F (190°C).
2. Take a large bowl and add in gram flour, corn flour, chilies, coriander leaves, salt, pepper, cumin powder, cinnamon powder, dry coriander powder, turmeric powder, and baking soda. Mix well.
3. Add 1/4 cup of water to make a thick batter.
4. Set aside for 2-3 minutes.
5. Now drop a spoonful of batter into air fryer basket at 1 inch apart from each other.
6. Let to cook for 8 minutes.
7. Serve and enjoy!

Nutrition Facts (Per Serving)

- Energy (calories): 75 kcal
- Protein: 3.68 g
- Fat: 1.2 g
- Carbohydrates: 12.48 g
- Dietary Fiber 2.1 g

Mixed Herb Fried Potatoes

Make these mix herb flavored potatoes and drizzle some lemon juice on top to enhance flavors. Enjoy this delight as your side dish proudly.

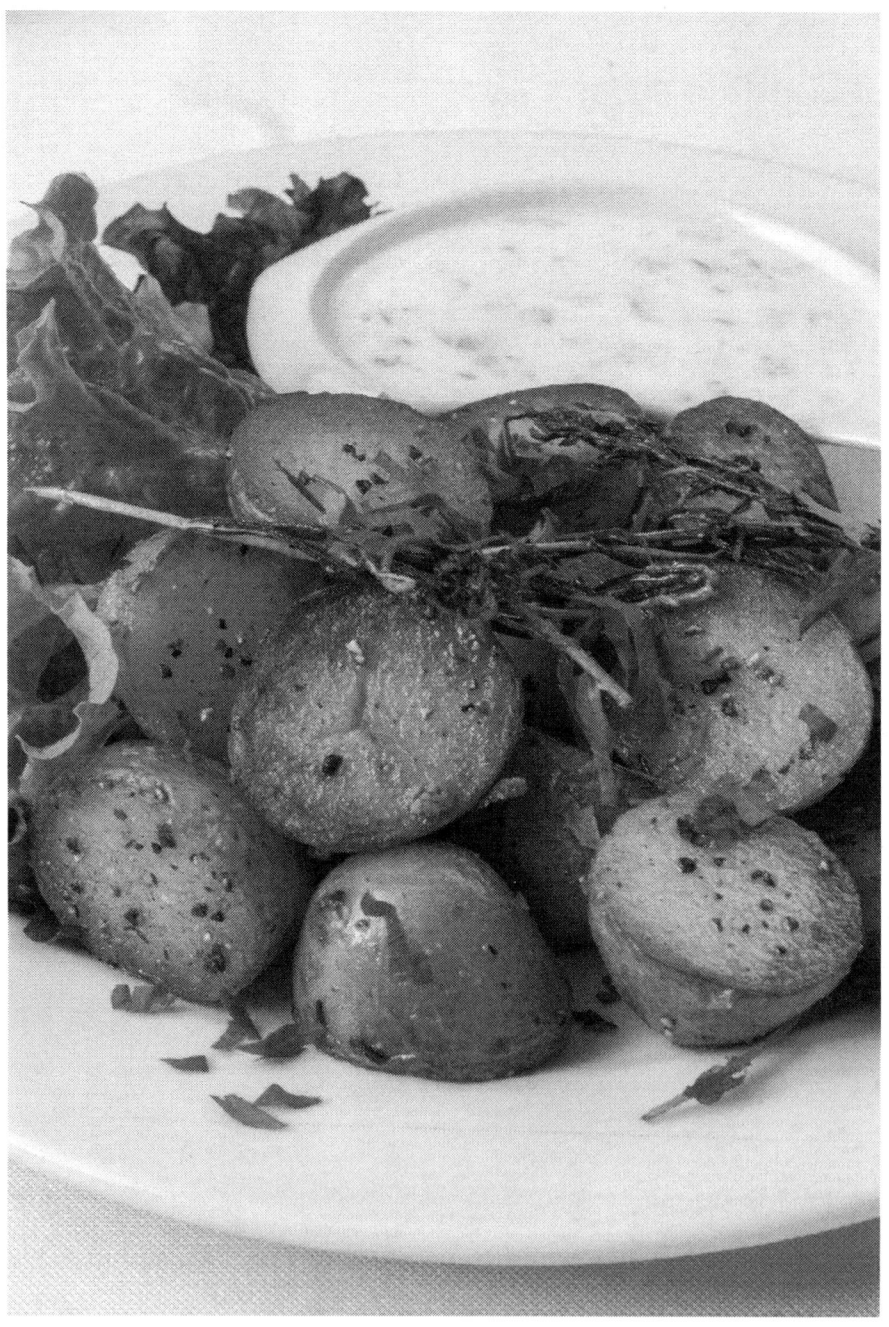

Serving: 4

Prep Time: 1 minute

Cook Time: 12 minutes

Ingredients

- 4-5 potatoes, diced
- 1 tablespoons mixed herbs
- ½ teaspoon cinnamon powder
- ¼ teaspoon cumin powder
- ¼ teaspoon dry coriander powder
- 1 tablespoons wheat flour
- 2 teaspoon olive oil
- ½ teaspoon salt
- ¼ teaspoon black pepper
- 1 teaspoon lemon juice

How To

1. In a bowl add potatoes, salt, mixed herbs, black pepper, olive oil, cumin powder, cinnamon powder, dry coriander powder, and wheat flour, toss well to combine.
2. Preheat your Air Fryer to a temperature of 380°F (190°C).
3. Put potatoes in air fryer basket and let them cook for 12 minutes.
4. Sake fryer basket after every 2 minutes.
5. When done transfer into serving the dish and drizzle lemon juice on top.
6. Serve!

Nutrition Facts (Per Serving)

- Energy (calories): 349 kcal
- Protein: 8.65 g
- Fat: 2.68 g
- Carbohydrates: 74.54 g
- Dietary Fiber 9.4 g

Crunchy Zucchini Chips

Make tempting zucchini chips for your kids and family members and surprise everyone. This is a perfect treat for your whole family.

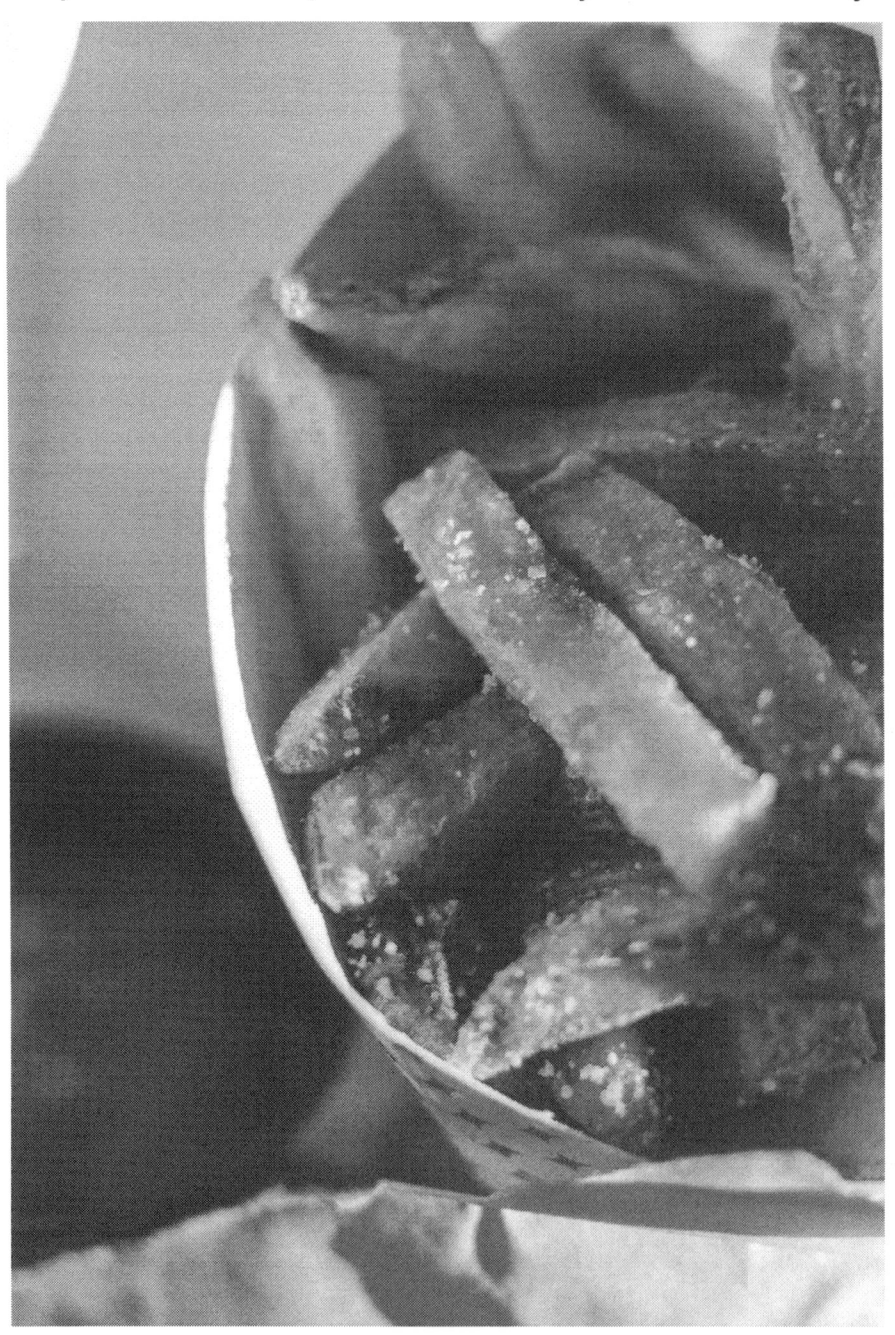

Serving: 4

Prep Time: 1 minute

Cook Time: 8 minutes

Ingredients

- 4 zucchinis, cut into chips
- 3 tablespoons gram flour
- ¼ teaspoon salt
- ¼ teaspoon chili powder
- ¼ teaspoon cumin powder

How To

1. Preheat your Air Fryer to a temperature of 320°F (160°C).
2. In a bowl add zucchini chips, salt, chili powder, and cumin powder, toss well to combine.
3. Transfer chips in air fryer basket and leave to cook for 8 minutes.
4. Shake fryer basket after every 2 minutes.
5. Serve and enjoy!

Nutrition Facts (Per Serving)

- Energy (calories): 51 kcal
- Protein: 3.39 g
- Fat: 0.97 g
- Carbohydrates: 8.74 g
- Dietary Fiber 2.5 g

Grated Potato Fritters

Make your friend and family happy with this quick and delicious snack. You have to grab potatoes and grate them. Roll them into gram flour batter and enjoy.

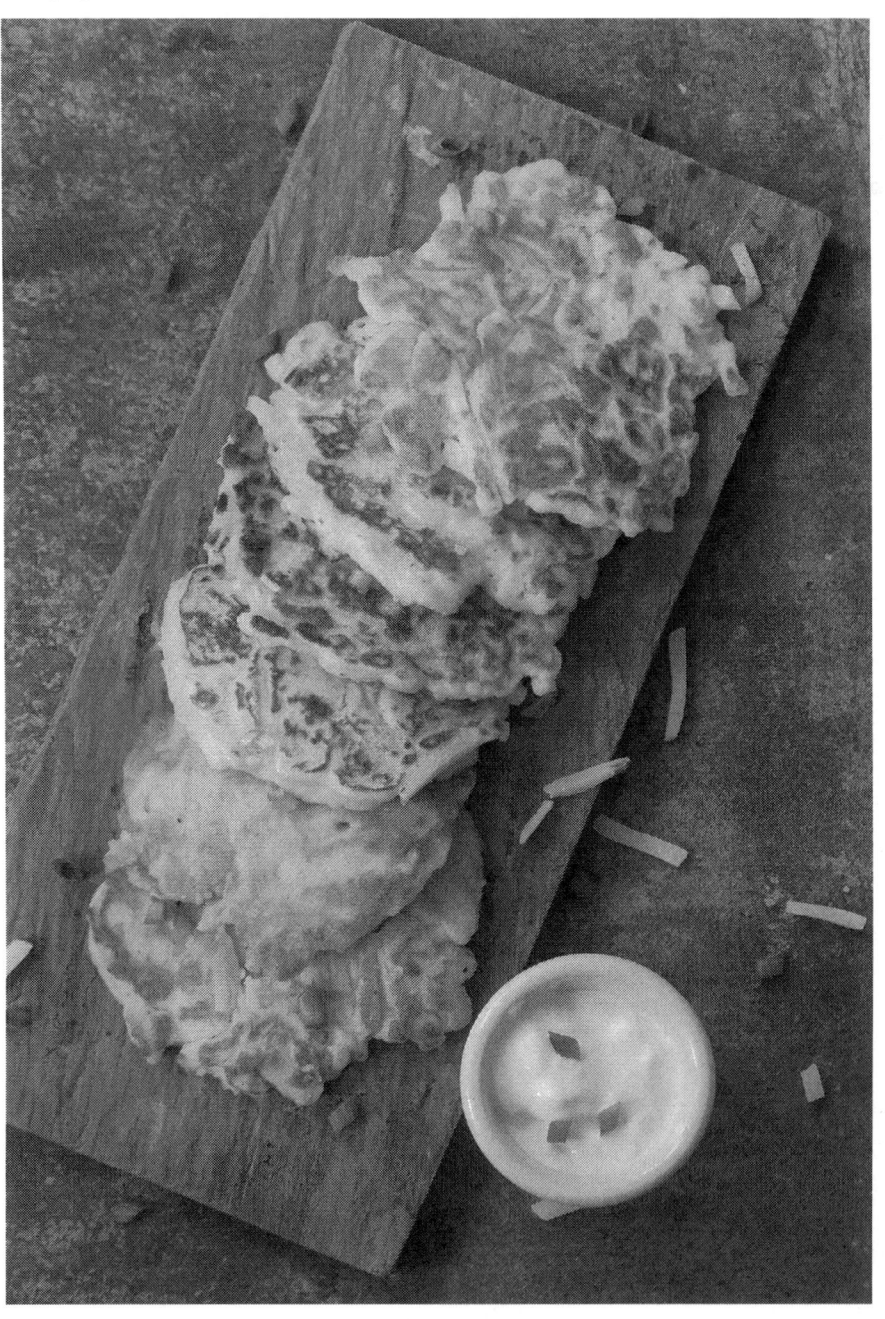

Serving: 6

Prep Time: 3 minutes

Cook Time: 8 minutes

Ingredients

- 4 potatoes, grated
- 1 cup gram flour
- ½ teaspoon chili powder
- ¼ teaspoon cumin powder
- ¼ teaspoon cinnamon powder
- ¼ teaspoon dry coriander powder
- 2 tablespoons coriander leaves, chopped
- ¼ teaspoon salt

How To

1. In a bowl add gram flour, salt, chili powder, cumin powder, cinnamon powder, dry coriander powder, and coriander leaves, mix well.
2. Add water and make a thick paste.
3. Now add potatoes and stir to combine.
4. Preheat Air Fryer at the temperature of 360°F (180°C).
5. Place 1 tablespoon of mixture into air fryer basket and leave to cook for 8 minutes.
6. Serve!

Nutrition Facts (Per Serving)

- Energy (calories): 163 kcal
- Protein: 6.11 g
- Fat: 1.16 g
- Carbohydrates: 32.58 g
- Dietary Fiber 4.7 g

Masala Roasted Potato Wedges

These crunch and spicy potatoes are going to give you a unique and enchanting taste that you never had before.

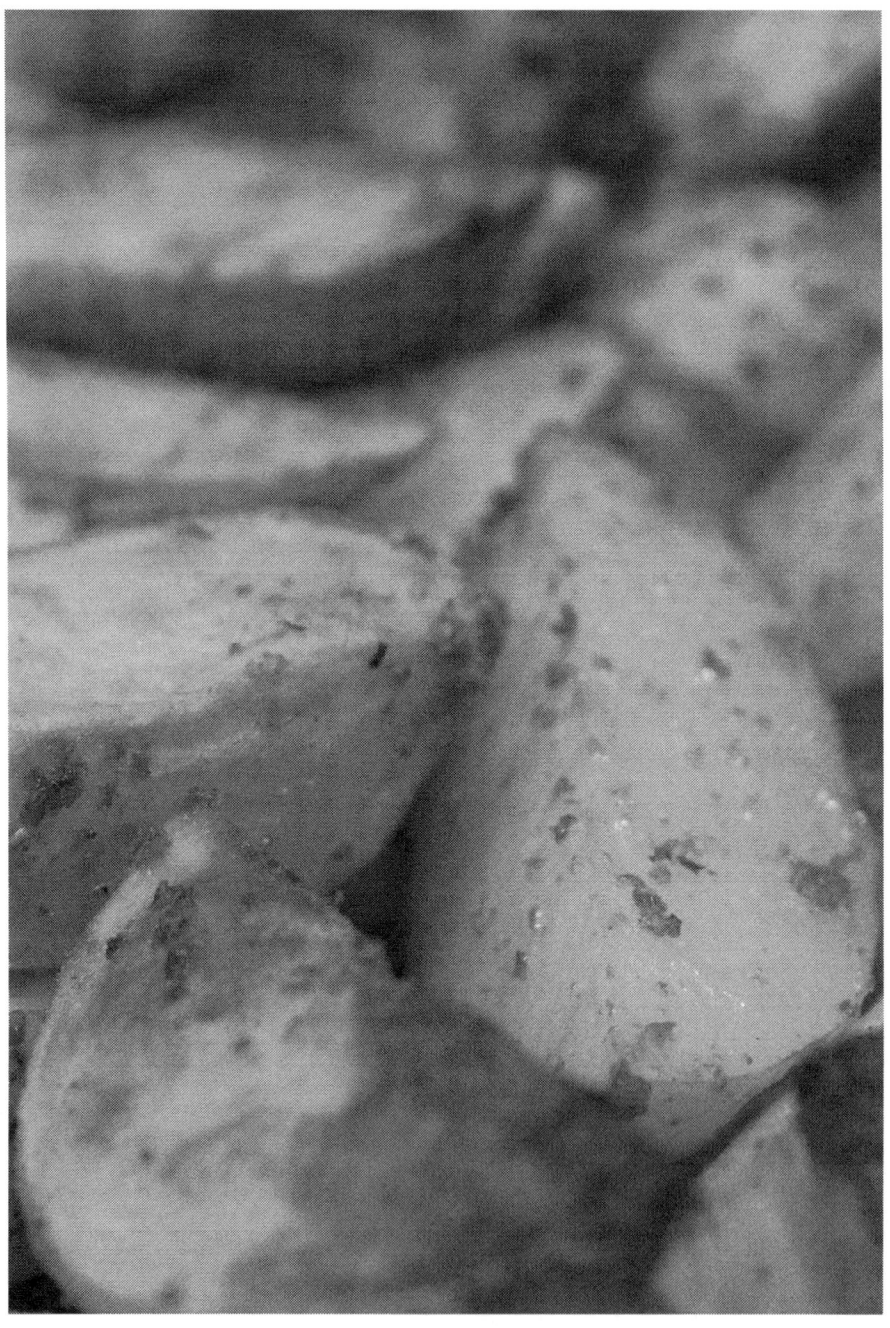

Serving: 4

Prep Time: 2 minutes

Cook Time: 12 minutes

Ingredients

- 4 potatoes, cut into wedges
- ¼ teaspoon chili powder
- ¼ teaspoon black pepper
- ¼ teaspoon cumin powder
- ¼ teaspoon cinnamon powder
- ¼ teaspoon dry mango powder
- ¼ teaspoon salt
- ¼ teaspoon dry coriander powder
- 3 tablespoons corn flour
- 1 pinch turmeric powder
- 1 teaspoon olive oil

How To

1. Preheat your Air Fryer to a temperature of 320°F (160°C).
2. In a large bowl add all spices, olive oil, and flour, mix well.
3. Add in potato wedges and toss well to coat.
4. Transfer potato wedges into air fryer basket and leave them to cook for 12 minutes.
5. Shake air fryer basket after 2 minutes.
6. Serve and enjoy!

Nutrition Facts (Per Serving)

- Energy (calories): 213 kcal
- Protein: 4.99 g
- Fat: 1.7 g
- Carbohydrates: 46.06 g
- Dietary Fiber 5.8 g

Roasted Peanuts

These peanuts are roasted with soya sauce, maple syrup, brown sugar and salt mixture. Will satisfy your taste buds and is the best solution for your carvings.

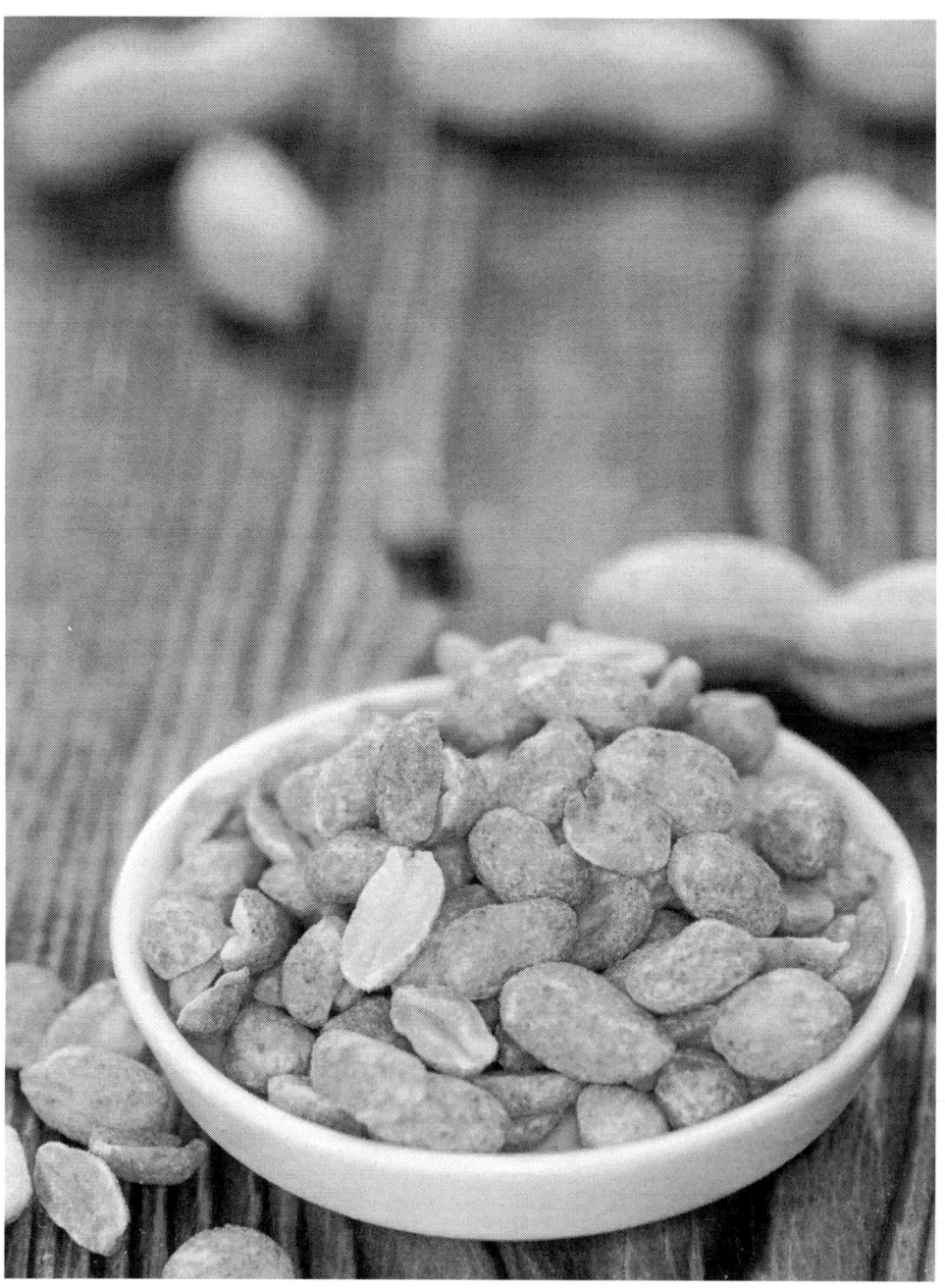

Serving: 4

Prep Time: 1 minute

Cook Time: 4 minutes

Ingredients

- 2 cups peanuts
- 1 tablespoon soya sauce
- 4 tablespoons brown sugar
- ¼ teaspoon salt
- 2 tablespoons maple syrup

How To

1. In a bow add peanuts, maple syrup, salt, brown sugar, and soya sauce, toss well to coat.
2. Preheat your Air Fryer to a temperature of 360°F (180°C).
3. Put peanuts into air fryer basket and let to cook for 4 minutes.
4. Shake basket after 2 minutes.
5. Serve with coffee or tea!

Nutrition Facts (Per Serving)

- Energy (calories): 484 kcal
- Protein: 18.43 g
- Fat: 34.74 g
- Carbohydrates: 33.05 g
- Dietary Fiber 6.5 g

Roasted Broccoli

These roasted broccolis are extremely delicious and healthy. You will love this simple and tempting dish surely.

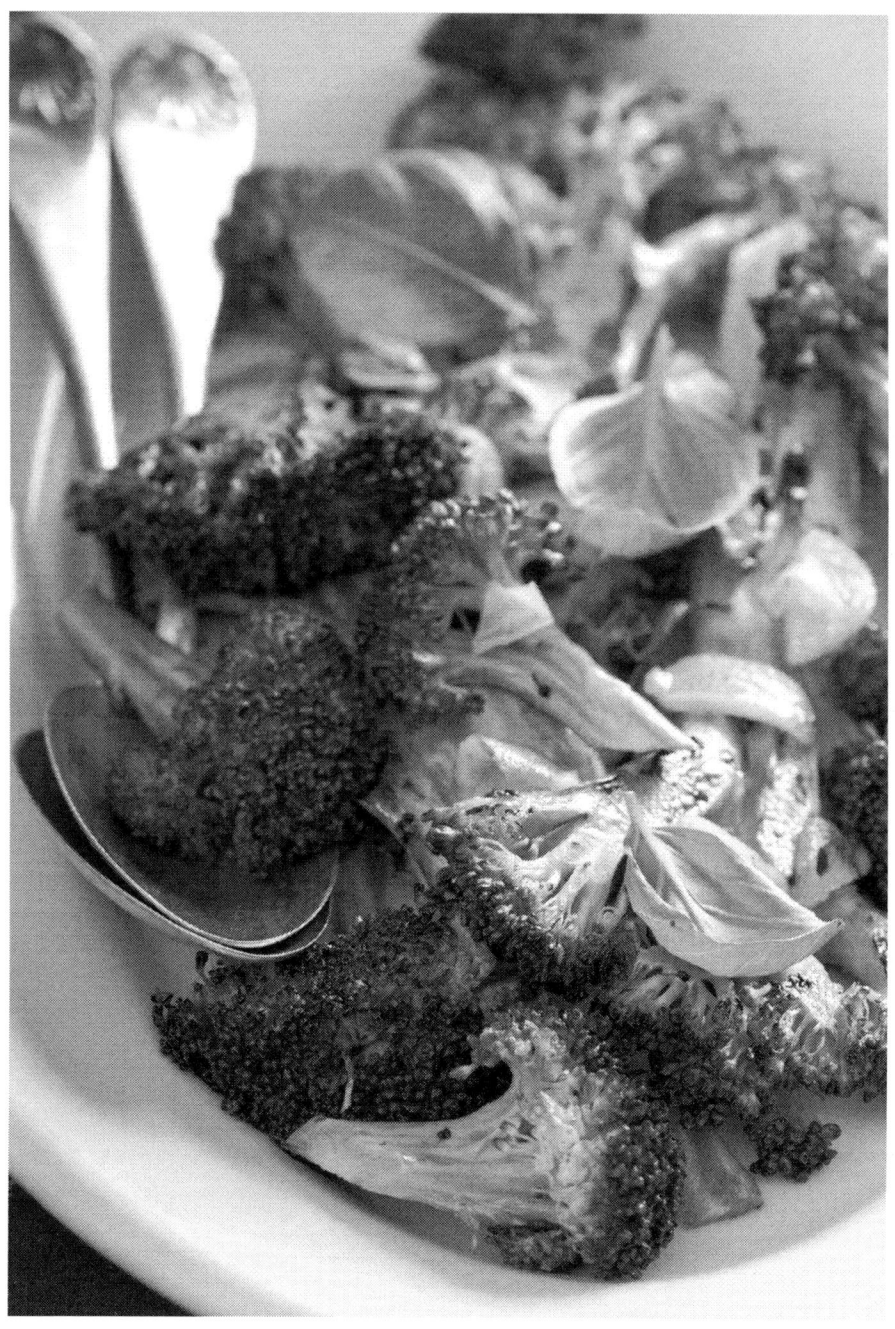

Serving: 2

Prep Time: 1 minute

Cook Time: 4 minutes

Ingredients

- 1-pound broccoli, florets
- 1 teaspoon black pepper
- ¼ teaspoon salt
- 1 teaspoon olive oil

How To

1. Sprinkle salt and black pepper on broccoli.
2. Drizzle olive oil on top and toss to combine.
3. Preheat your Air Fryer to a temperature of 380°F (190°C).
4. Put broccoli florets in air fryer basket and cook for 4 minutes.
5. Shake basket after 2 minutes so that all florets can cook evenly.
6. Serve!

Nutrition Facts (Per Serving)

- Energy (calories): 73 kcal
- Protein: 7.34 g
- Fat: 3.41 g
- Carbohydrates: 7.39 g
- Dietary Fiber 6.5 g

Air Fried Crispy Chili Bites

These oil fewer chili bits are made up of gram flour, onion, green chilies, fresh coriander leaves, and mint leaves. Your kid will love these bites.

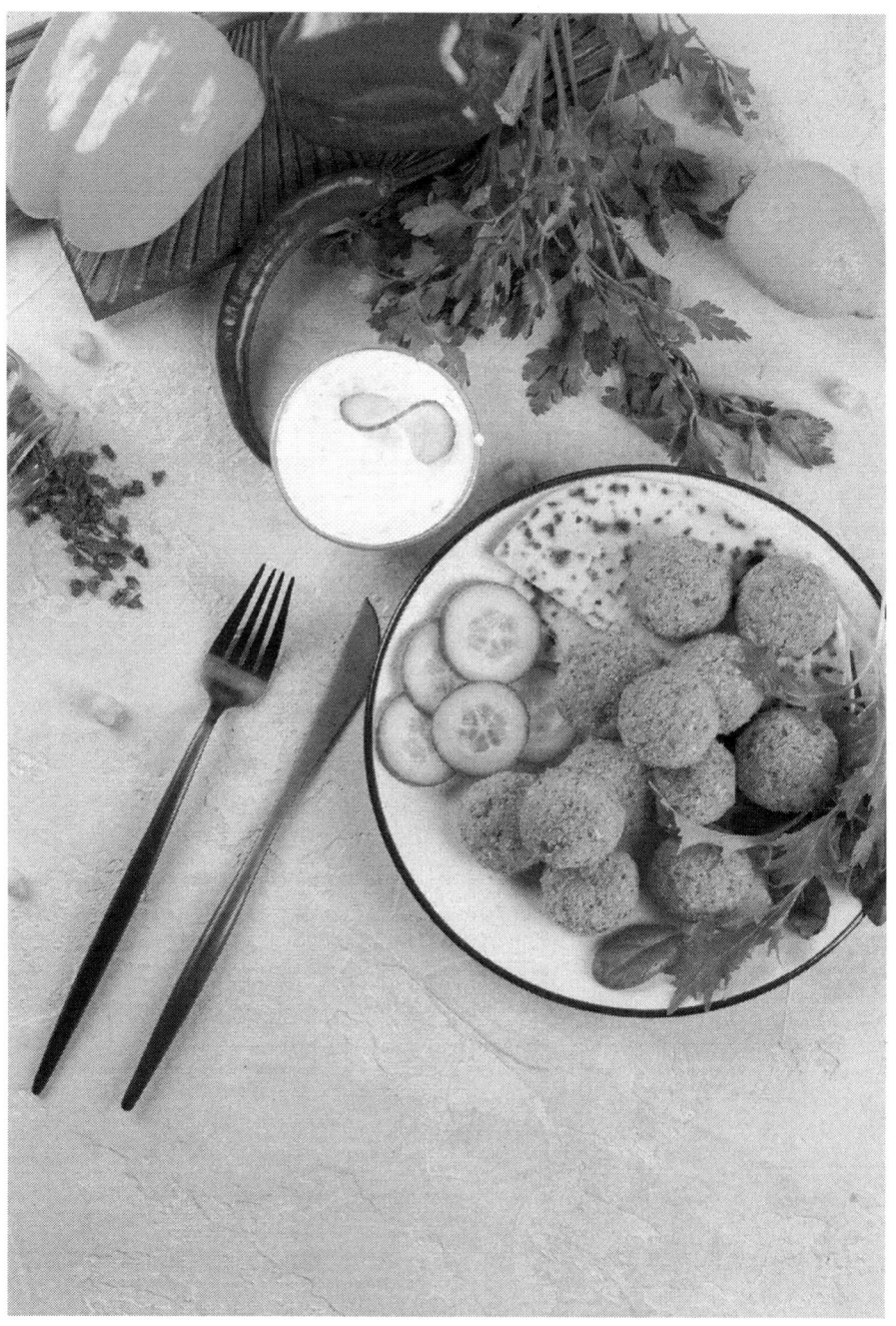

Serving: 6

Prep Time: 2 minutes

Cook Time: 8 minutes

Ingredients

- 1 cup gram flour
- 2 onions, thinly sliced
- 3-4 green chilies, chopped
- 1 bunch mint leaves, chopped
- 1 bunch coriander leaves, chopped
- ¼ teaspoon salt
- ¼ teaspoon cinnamon powder
- ¼ teaspoon cumin powder

How To

1. In a bowl add gram flour, onion, chilies, salt, coriander leaves, mint leaves, cinnamon powder, and cumin powder, mix well.
2. Now add ¼ cup of water and make a thick paste.
3. Preheat Air Fryer to a temperature of 360°F (180°C).
4. Drop one tablespoon of mixture into air fryer basket at ½ inch distance apart from each other.
5. Now leave to cook for 8 minutes.
6. Serve.

Nutrition Facts (Per Serving)

- Energy (calories): 97 kcal
- Protein: 5.5 g
- Fat: 1.63 g
- Carbohydrates: 15.03 g
- Dietary Fiber 3.1 g

Indian Style Kurkuri Lady Fingers

It's a unique and flavorful dish for all those who love to eat vegetables. It's the best way to add organic lady fingers to your diet.

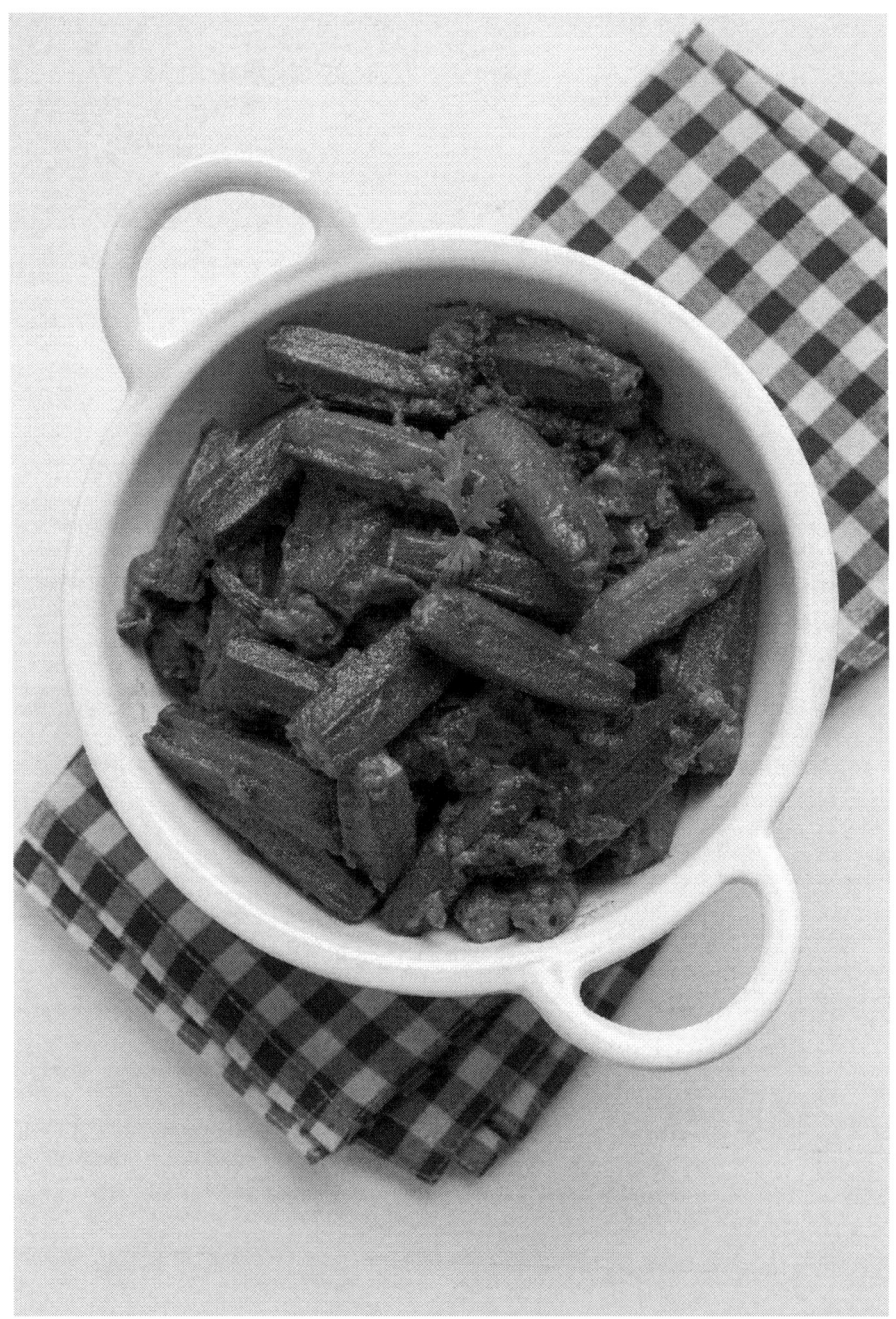

Serving: 4

Prep Time: 2 minutes

Cook Time: 8 minutes

Ingredients

- 1 ½ pound lady fingers (Okra)
- 4 tablespoons gram flour
- ½ teaspoon chili powder
- ½ teaspoon cinnamon powder
- ¼ teaspoon salt

How To

1. Preheat Air Fryer to a temperature of 380°F (190°C).
2. In a large bowl add ladyfingers and sprinkle gram flour, salt, chili powder and cinnamon powder on top, toss to coat well.
3. Put ladyfingers into air fryer basket and cook for 4 minutes.
4. Shake basket after 2 minutes.
5. Serve!

Nutrition Facts (Per Serving)

- Energy (calories): 62 kcal
- Protein: 3.45 g
- Fat: 0.39 g
- Carbohydrates: 13.87 g
- Dietary Fiber 5.8 g

Banana Wafers

If you are craving for a quick and tempting snack, then give a try to this dish. Serve them with yogurt dip and make happy yourself!

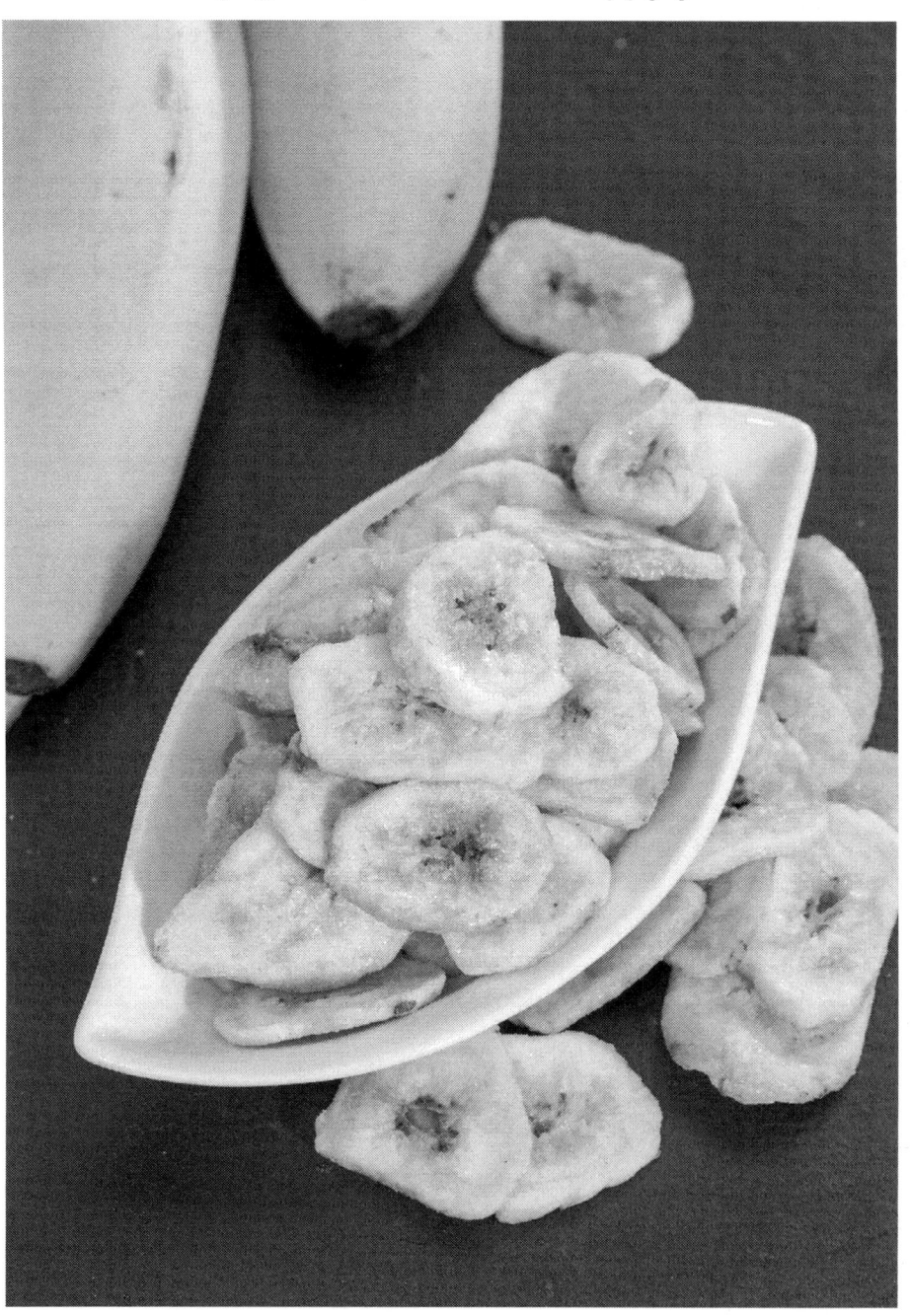

Serving: 4

Prep Time: 1 minute

Cook Time: 4 minutes

Ingredients

- 4 raw bananas, peeled, thinly sliced
- ¼ teaspoon salt
- ¼ teaspoon black pepper

How To

1. Sprinkle salt and black pepper on bananas
2. Preheat Air Fryer at the temperature of 360°F (180°C).
3. Put chips into air fryer basket and leave to cook for 4 minutes.
4. Serve and enjoy!

Nutrition Facts (Per Serving)

- Energy (calories): 121 kcal
- Protein: 1.5 g
- Fat: 0.45 g
- Carbohydrates: 31.17 g
- Dietary Fiber 3.6 g

Baked Turnip Chips

This is a unique dish for all those who love to have a quick and delicious snack, serve them with a hot and sour dip or mayo dip to enhance more flavors.

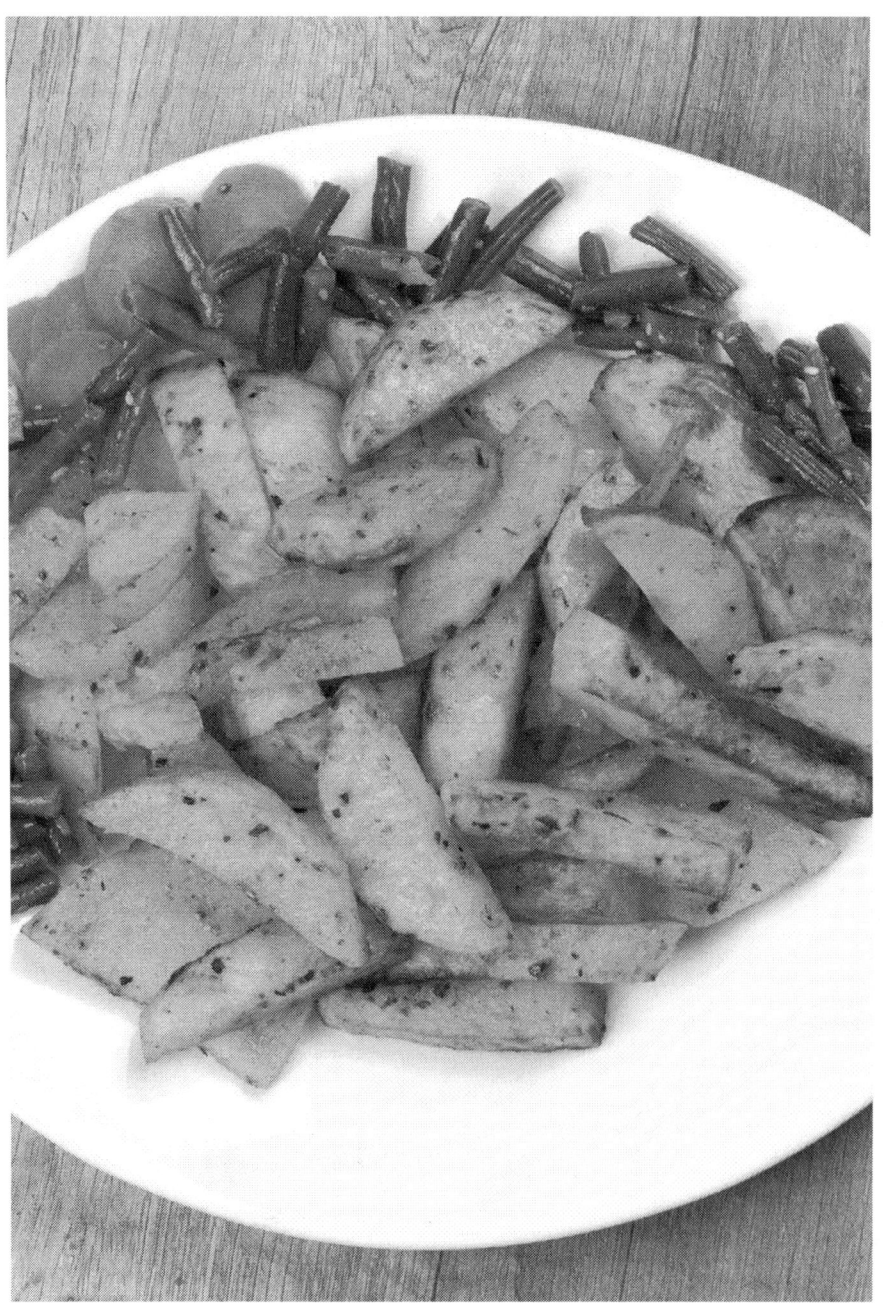

Serving: 4

Prep Time: 2 minutes

Cook Time: 8 minutes

Ingredients

- 4 turnips, peeled, cut into 1-inch slices
- ¼ teaspoon salt
- ¼ teaspoon chili flakes
- ¼ teaspoon black pepper
- 2 tablespoons vinegar

How To

1. Preheat your Air Fryer to a temperature of 320°F (160°C).
2. In a bowl add turnip chips, salt, pepper, chili flakes, and vinegar, toss well to combine.
3. Transfer in air fryer basket and cook for 8 minutes.
4. Shake basket after two every minute.
5. Serve and enjoy!

Nutrition Facts (Per Serving)

- Energy (calories): 54 kcal
- Protein: 1.69 g
- Fat: 0.21 g
- Carbohydrates: 12.04 g
- Dietary Fiber 3.4 g

Air Fried Crusty Baked Tofu

If you are looking for a tofu delight that can be cooked quickly then have this one. You will love to make these breadcrumb coated tofus.

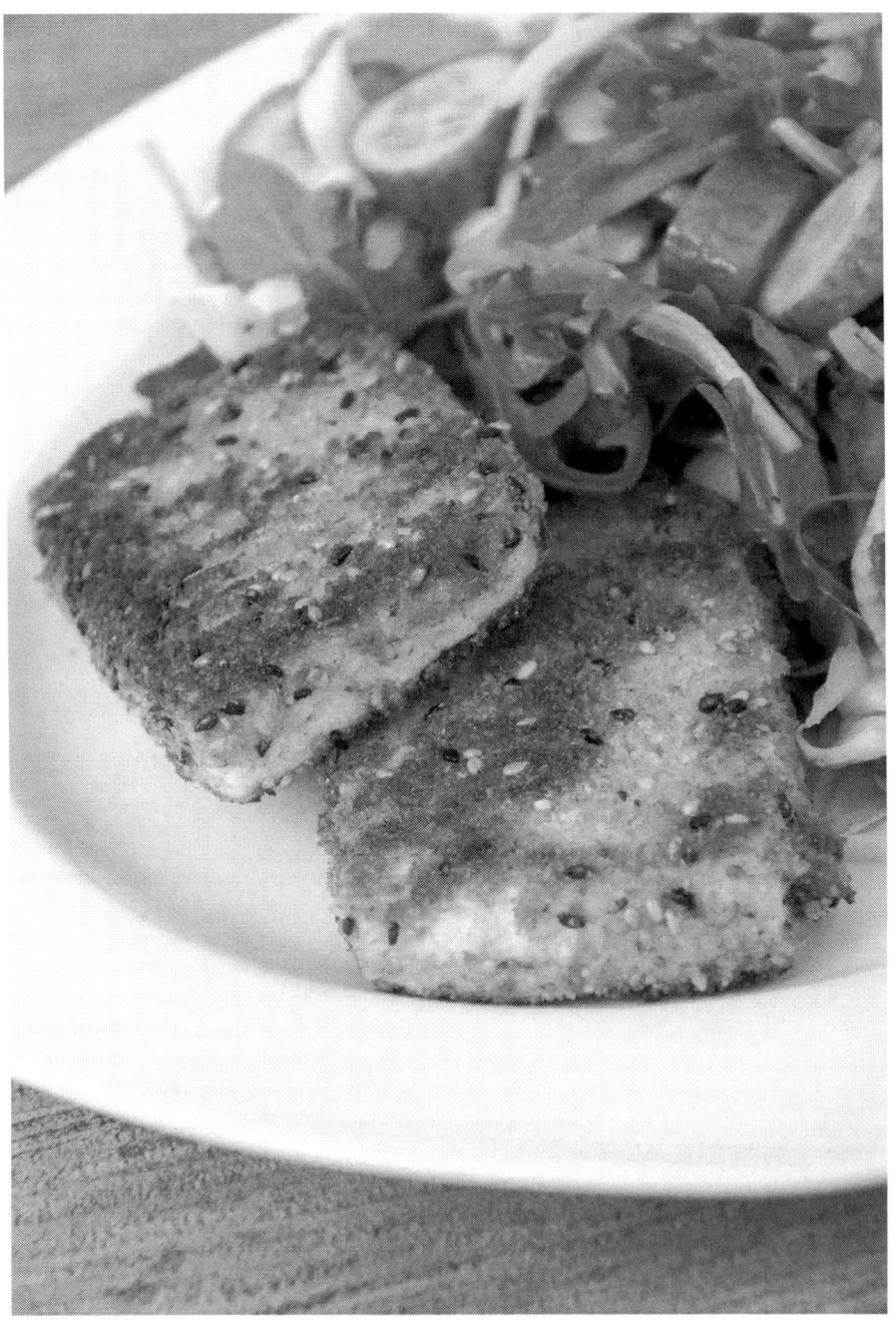

Serving: 4

Prep Time: 1 minute

Cook Time: 8 minutes

Ingredients

- 1 ½ pound tofu, cut into 2-inch slices
- ¼ teaspoon chili powder
- 1 tablespoon olive oil
- 1 teaspoon oregano
- ¼ teaspoon salt
- ¼ teaspoon garlic powder
- ½ tablespoon sesame

How To

1. In a bowl add breadcrumbs, salt, garlic powder, sesame, and oregano, mix well.
2. Brush tofu with olive and roll them into breadcrumbs mixture.
3. Sprinkle chili powder on the top of each tofu.
4. Preheat your Air Fryer to a temperature of 360°F (180°C).
5. Place tofu in air fryer basket and cook for 8 minutes.
6. Serve hot with salad.

Nutrition Facts (Per Serving)

- Energy (calories): 278 kcal
- Protein: 26.92 g
- Fat: 18.24 g
- Carbohydrates: 7.67 g
- Dietary Fiber 4.1 g

Roasted Cauliflower Bites

This dish is made up of cauliflower florets that are coated with cayenne pepper, chili flakes, turmeric powder, olive oil, garlic powder, salt, and lime juice mixture.

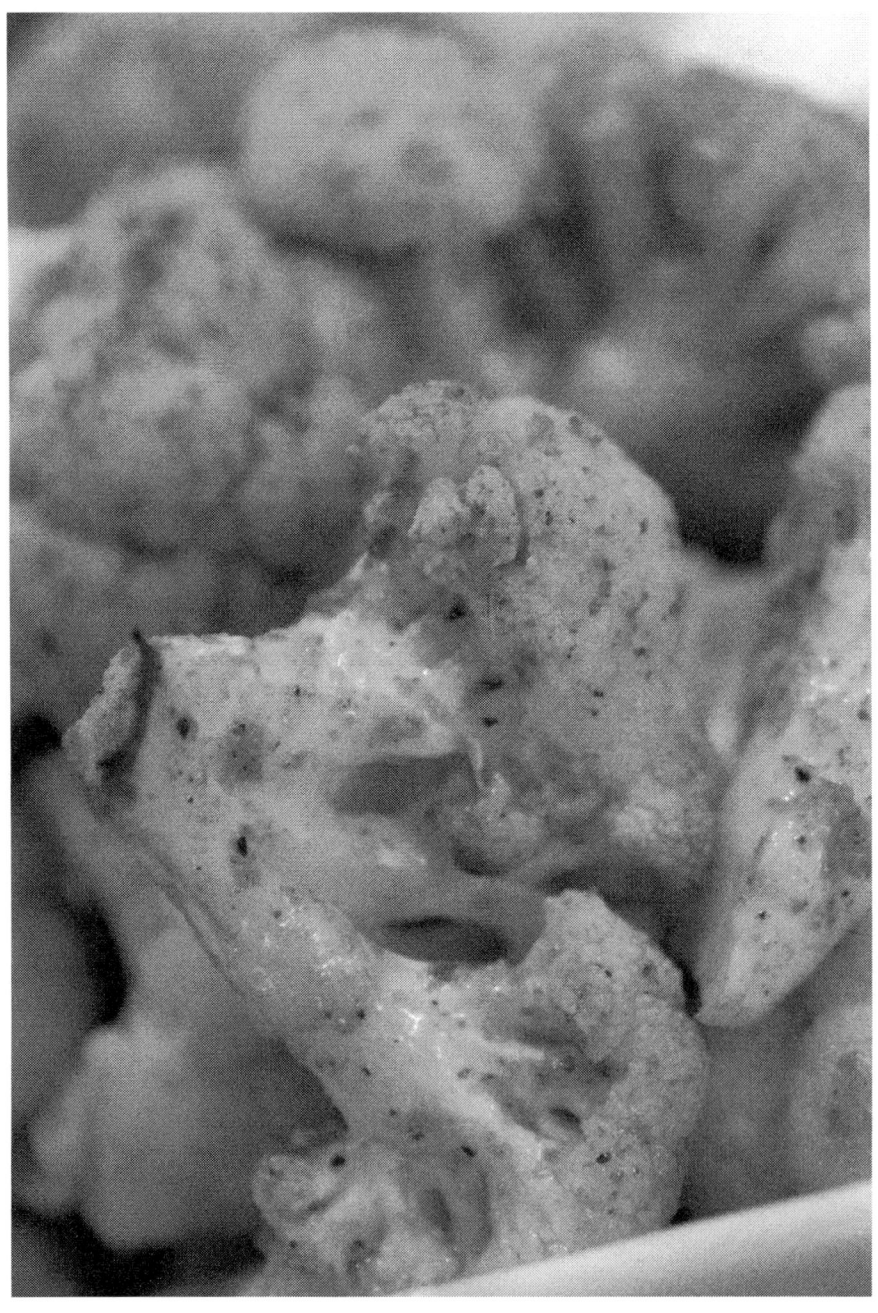

Serving: 4

Prep Time: 1 minute

Cook Time: 8 minutes

Ingredients

- 1-pound cauliflower florets
- ½ teaspoon cayenne pepper
- 1 pinch turmeric powder
- ¼ teaspoon garlic powder
- ¼ teaspoon chili flakes
- ¼ teaspoon salt
- 1 teaspoon olive oil 2 tablespoons lime juice

How To

1. In a large bowl add cauliflower florets, salt, chili flakes, cayenne pepper, turmeric powder, olive oil, garlic powder, and lime juice, mix well.
2. Preheat your Air Fryer to a temperature of 380°F (190°C).
3. Put all cauliflower florets in air fryer basket and cook for 8 minutes.
4. Serve.

Nutrition Facts (Per Serving)

- Energy (calories): 31 kcal
- Protein: 2.27 g
- Fat: 0.38 g
- Carbohydrates: 6.1 g
- Dietary Fiber 2.4 g

Crunchy Cucumber Chips

This is very easy and delicious recipe that everyone wants. Make your friend and family happy with this uniquely flavored and tempting delight.

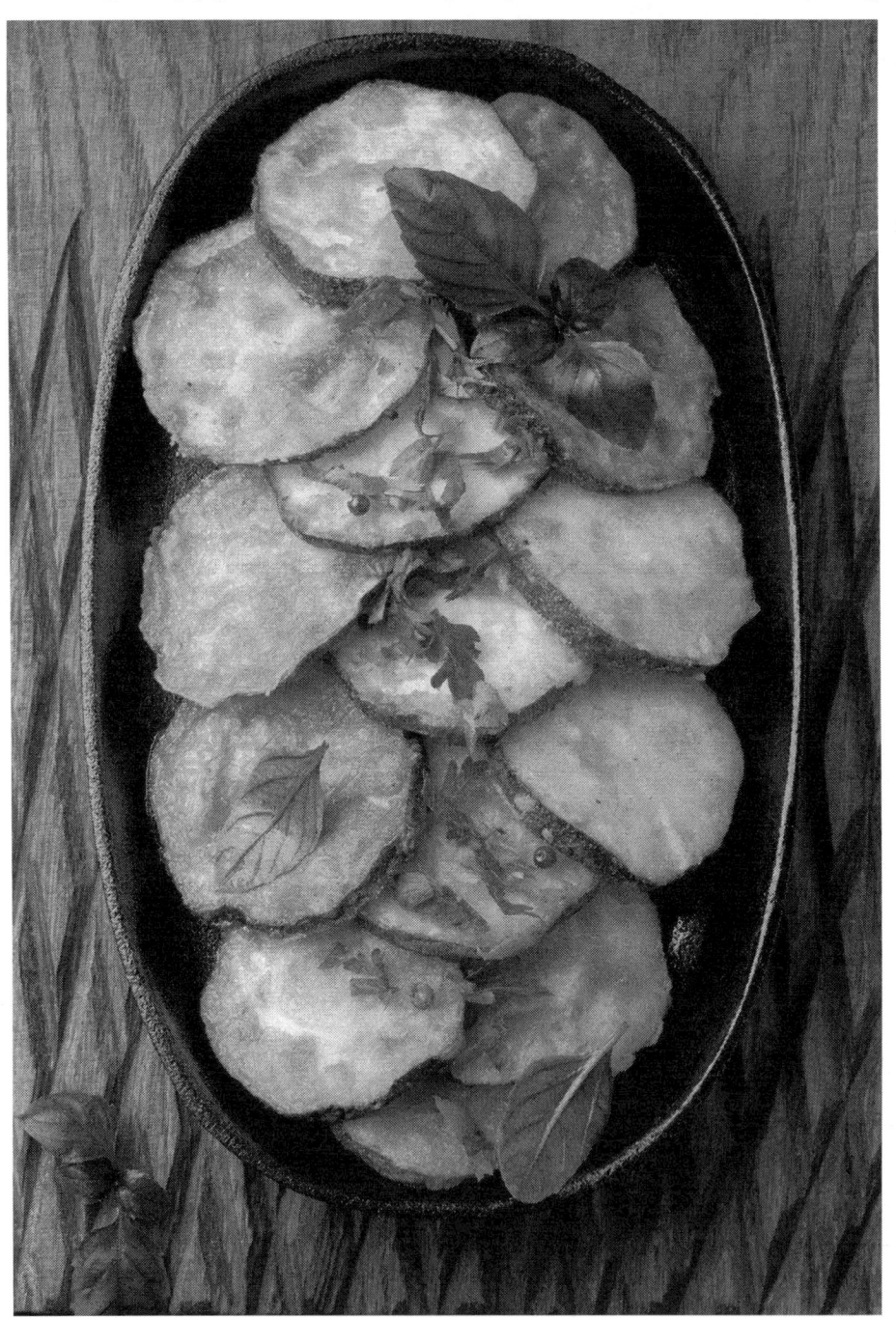

Serving: 4

Prep Time: 1 minute

Cook Time: 4 minutes

Ingredients

- 4 cucumbers, thinly sliced
- ¼ cup corn flour
- ¼ teaspoon garlic powder
- ¼ teaspoon salt
- 1 teaspoon caster sugar

How To

1. In a bowl add cucumber chips and sprinkle corn flour, salt, garlic powder, and caster sugar, mix to coat.
2. Preheat Air Fryer at the temperature of 380°F (190°C).
3. Put cucumber chips in air fryer basket and cook them for 4 minutes.
4. Shake fryer basket after 2 minutes so that they can cook evenly.
5. Bon Appetit!

Nutrition Facts (Per Serving)

- Energy (calories): 63 kcal
- Protein: 2.19 g
- Fat: 0.73 g
- Carbohydrates: 12.45 g
- Dietary Fiber 2.5 g

Roasted Potatoes, Brussels Sprouts, and Squash

This colorful dish is made with potatoes and squash and flavored with some ginger powder, coconut oil, and black pepper.

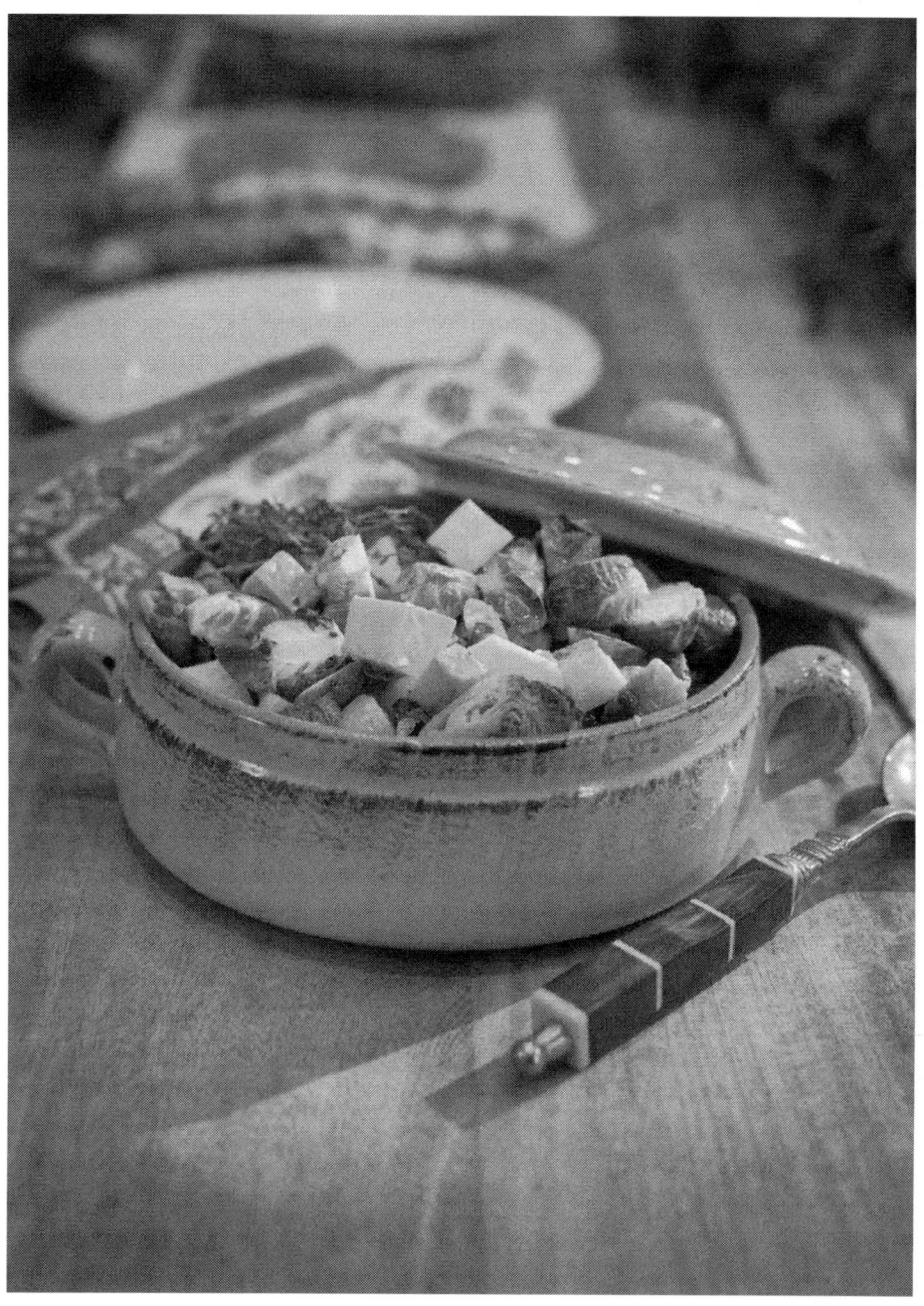

Serving: 4

Prep Time: 2 minutes

Cook Time: 12 minutes

Ingredients

- 3 potatoes, cut into small cubes
- ½ pound squash, cut into small cubes
- ½ pound Brussels sprouts
- ¼ teaspoon ginger powder
- Salt and black pepper, to taste
- 2 tablespoons coconut oil

How To

1. Preheat Air Fryer at a temperature of 360°F (180°C).
2. Sprinkle ginger powder, salt and black pepper on potatoes, Brussels sprouts, and squash.
3. Drizzle coconut oil and toss to combine.
4. Transfer potatoes, Brussels sprouts, and squash into fryer basket and leave to cook for 12 minutes.
5. Shake fryer basket after every 2 minutes.
6. Serve.

Nutrition Facts (Per Serving)

- Energy (calories): 232 kcal
- Protein: 4.3 g
- Fat: 7.09 g
- Carbohydrates: 40.86 g
- Dietary Fiber 5.4 g

Fresh Bean Fries

These fresh beans are pickled in vinegar and soya sauce and cooked in air fryer for only 8 minutes. You can add sugar if you want a sweet and sour taste.

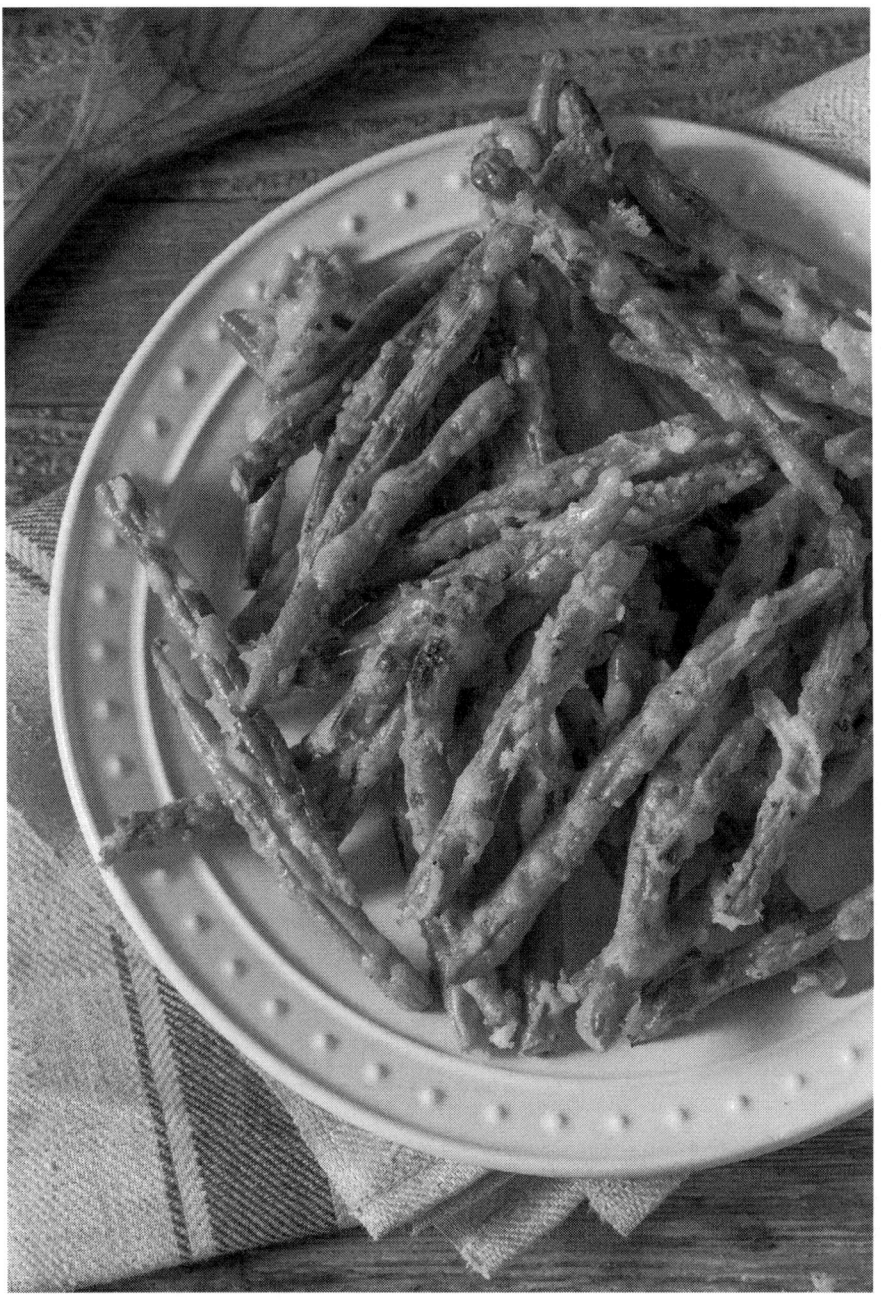

Serving: 2

Prep Time: 30 minutes

Cook Time: 8 minutes

Ingredients

- 1-pound fresh beans
- ½ cup vinegar
- ¼ teaspoon salt
- 3 tablespoons soya sauce

How To

1. In a large bowl add fresh beans, salt, vinegar, and soya sauce, mix well and place aside for 30 minutes.
2. Preheat your Air Fryer to a temperature of 320°F (160°C).
3. Now transfer fresh beans into air fryer basket and cook for 8 minutes.
4. Shake fryer basket after 4 minutes.
5. Put to serving platter when done.
6. Serve and enjoy.

Nutrition Facts (Per Serving)

- Energy (calories): 70 kcal
- Protein: 2.96 g
- Fat: 1.09 g
- Carbohydrates: 12.17 g
- Dietary Fiber 4.8 g

Baked Baisan Roti

This is the best option for those who want a different dish for their daily routine. You can preserve these roties for later use also.

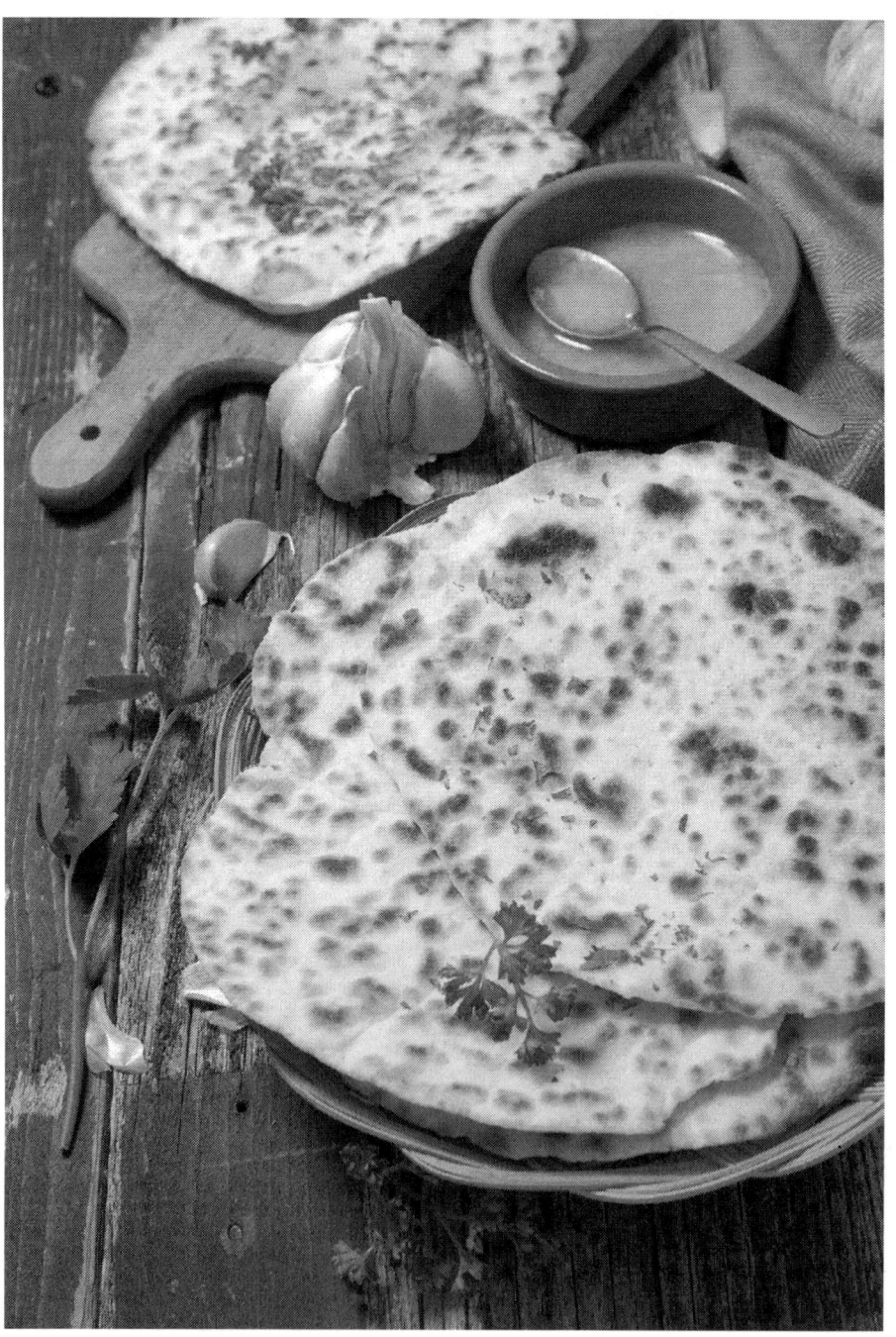

Serving: 4

Prep Time: 15 minutes

Cook Time: 4 minutes

Ingredients

- 1 cup gram flour
- ¼ cup wheat flour
- 1 tablespoon butter, melted
- 1 bunch coriander leaves, chopped
- ¼ teaspoon cumin powder
- ¼ teaspoon salt
- ¼ teaspoon chili powder
- 1 pinch turmeric powder

How To

1. Take a bowl and add gram flour, wheat flour, salt, chili powder, turmeric powder, cumin powder, and coriander leaves, mix well.
2. Add some water and knead a soft dough.
3. Cover dough with a plastic wrap and set aside for 15 minutes.
4. Now make 4-5 round balls with the dough and roll each into a thin sheet.
5. Preheat your Air Fryer to a temperature of 360°F (180°C).
6. Place one sheet into air fryer basket at once, leave to cook for 4 minutes. Make all roties with the same way.
7. When done remove from air fryer basket and brush them with butter.
8. Serve with tea.

Nutrition Facts (Per Serving)

- Energy (calories): 144 kcal
- Protein: 6.03 g
- Fat: 4.55 g
- Carbohydrates: 19.41 g
- Dietary Fiber 2.8 g

Dal Moong Pakoras

These dal pakoras are made up of yellow lentil that is soaked in water for 4-5 hours and combined with chilies, coriander leaves, mint leaves, and some spices.

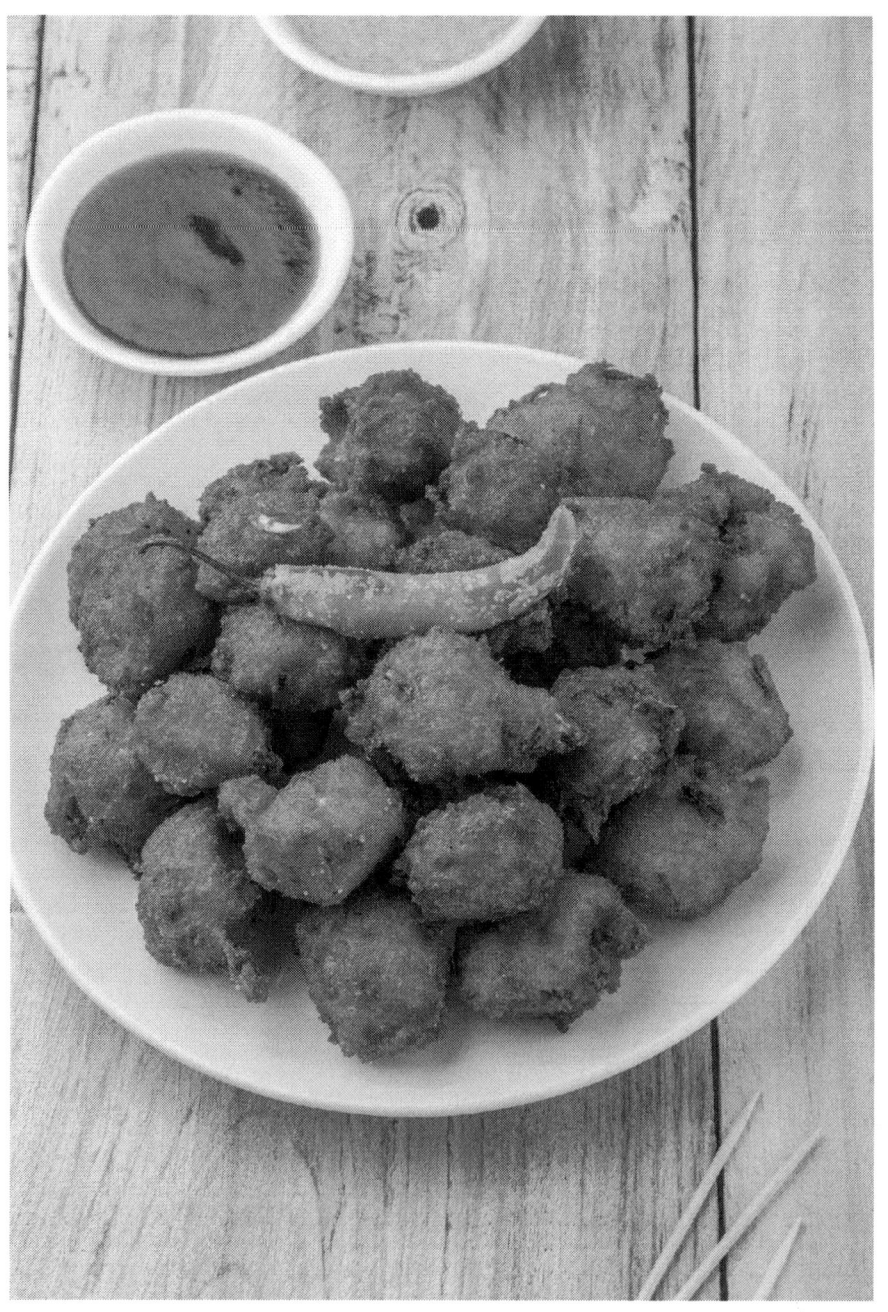

Serving: 5

Prep Time: 4 hours

Cook Time: 8 minutes

Ingredients

- 1 ½ cup yellow lentil, soaked in water for 4 hours
- 1 bunch coriander leaves, chopped
- 2 tablespoons mint leaves, chopped
- 2 green chilies
- 1-2 garlic cloves
- ¼ teaspoon salt
- ¼ teaspoon chili powder
- ¼ teaspoon cumin powder
- ¼ teaspoon cinnamon powder
- ¼ teaspoon baking powder

How To

1. Soak yellow lentils in the water for 4-5 hours
2. In a food processor add yellow lentil, coriander, mint, chilies, salt, chili powder, garlic, cumin powder, cinnamon powder, and baking powder, blend until pureed.
3. Preheat your Air Fryer to a temperature of 380°F (190°C).
4. Now place a tablespoon of mixture into air fryer basket at a distance apart from each other.
5. Leave pakoras to cook for 8 minutes.
6. Serve.

Nutrition Facts (Per Serving)

- Energy (calories): 60 kcal
- Protein: 3.66 g
- Fat: 0.47 g
- Carbohydrates: 12.28 g
- Dietary Fiber 1.7 g

Cinnamon Rolled Banana Bites

These banana bites are made up with banana slices rolled into cinnamon and maple syrup mixture. Your kids will fall in love with them.

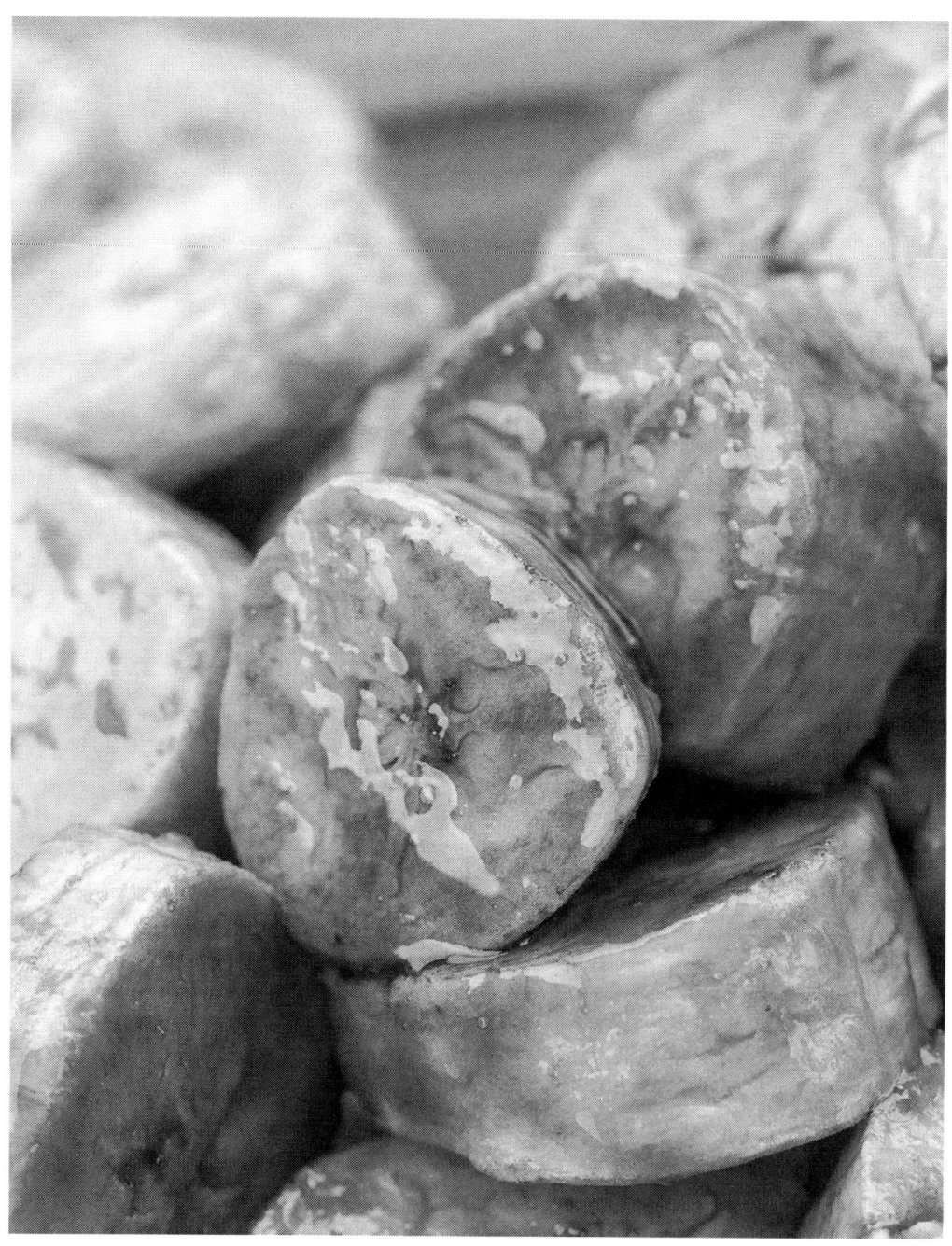

Serving: 4

Prep Time: 2 minutes

Cook Time: 8 minutes

Ingredients

- 4 large bananas, cut into ½ inch thick slices
- 4 tablespoons cinnamon powder
- ½ cup maple syrup
- ¼ teaspoon vanilla essences
- 1 tablespoon icing sugar

How To

1. Preheat Air Fryer at a temperature of 360°F (180°C).
2. In a bowl add maple syrup and vanilla essence, mix well.
3. Dip each banana slice into maple syrup mixture and roll out into cinnamon.
4. Place each banana slice into air fryer basket and leave to cook for 8 minutes.
5. Shake after half time so that they can cook evenly.
6. Transfer into serving platter and dust with icing sugar.

Nutrition Facts (Per Serving)

- Energy (calories): 278 kcal
- Protein: 1.92
- Fat: 0.55 g
- Carbohydrates: 74.3 g
- Dietary Fiber: 7.8g

Roasted Pineapples with Vanilla Zest

If you are trying to make a delicious and easy dessert, then this recipe is a sure try. It will need just a few minutes to make. Serve immediately when done.

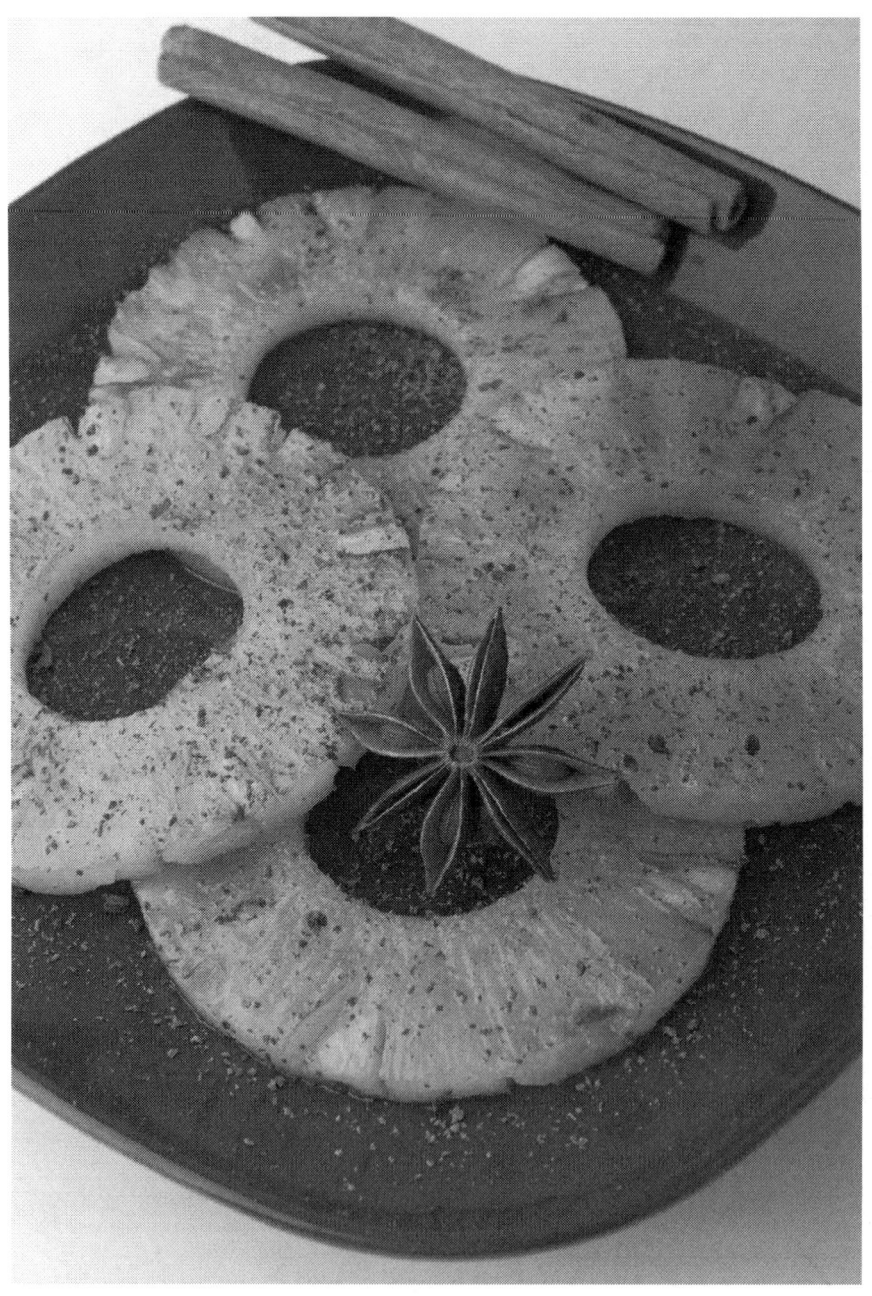

Servings: 4

Prep Time: 5 minutes

Cook Time: 8 minutes

Ingredients

- 1-pound pineapple slices
- 2 tablespoons caster sugar
- ¼ cup pineapple juice
- ¼ cup orange juice
- 2 anise stars
- 1 vanilla pod
- 1 teaspoon lime juice

How To

1. Preheat Air Fryer to a temperature of 360°F (180°C).
2. Take a baking pan that can fit into Air Fryer basket.
3. Now add pineapple juice, sugar, orange juice, anise stars, and vanilla pod into a pan and mix well.
4. Place in pineapple slices evenly and transfer pan into Air Fryer basket.
5. Cook for 8 minutes.
6. Serve.

Nutrition Facts (Per Serving)

- Energy (calories): 90 kcal
- Protein: 0.79 g
- Fat: 0.17 g
- Carbohydrates: 23.22 g
- Dietary Fiber: 1.8 g

Air Fryer Baked Apples

These baked apples are stuffed with maple syrup, brown sugar, raisins, and crushed walnuts. This exquisite delicacy melts in your mouth. You will love baked apples cooked in your Air fryer.

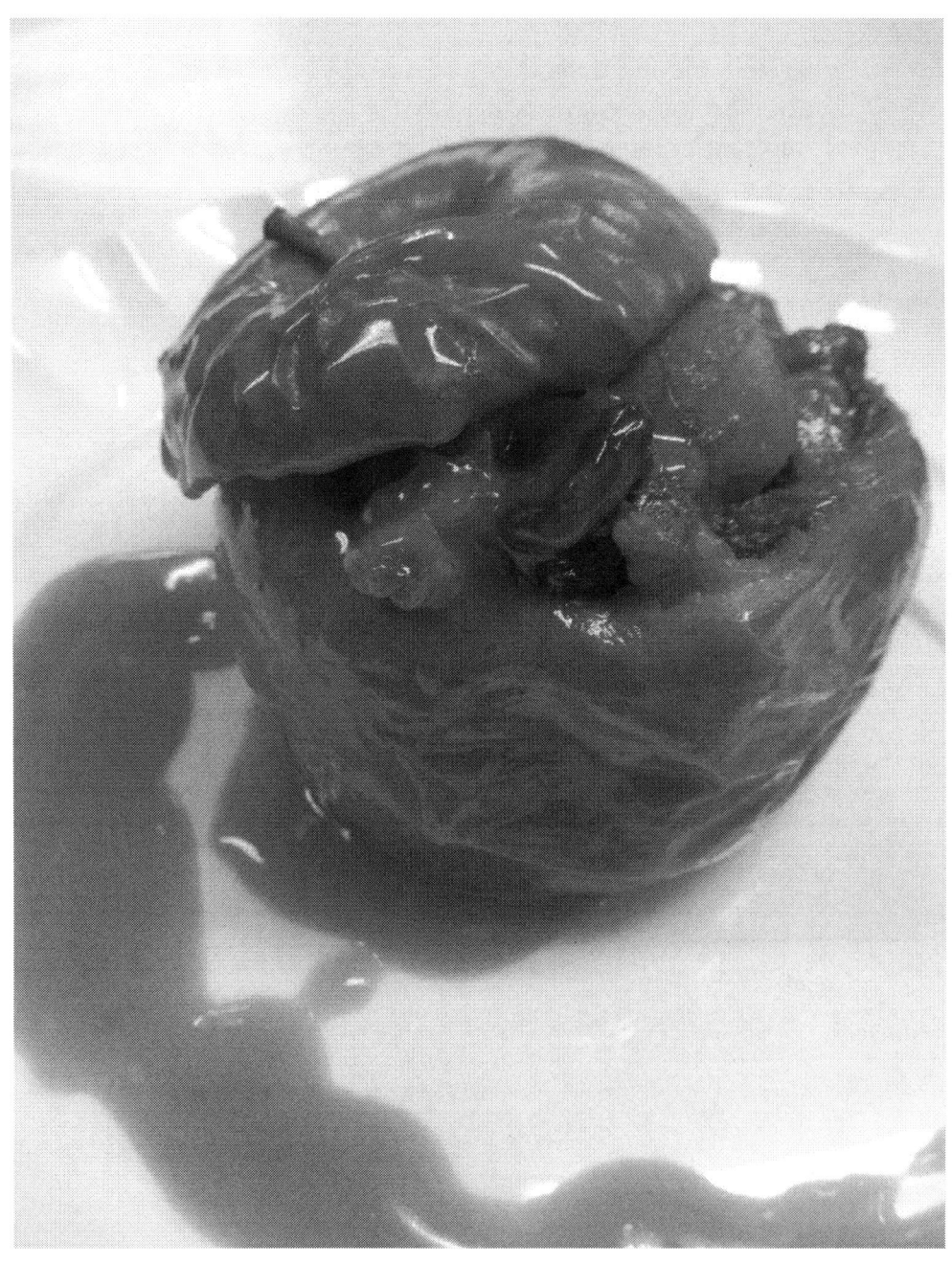

Servings: 4

Prep Time: 3 minutes

Cook Time: 12 minutes

Ingredients

- 4 large apples
- ¼ cup brown sugar
- 4 tablespoons maple syrup or sugar
- ½ cup walnuts, crushed
- ½ cup raisins

How To

1. Preheat Air Fryer to a temperature of 360°F (180°C).
2. Cut the apples from the stem and remove the inner using spoon.
3. Now fill each apple with raisins, walnuts, maple syrup, and brown sugar.
4. Transfer apples in a pan and place in Air Fryer basket, cook for 12 minutes.
5. Serve.

Nutrition Facts (Per Serving)

- Energy (calories): 324 kcal
- Protein: 2.8 g
- Fat: 6.99 g
- Carbohydrates: 70.31 g
- Dietary Fiber: 6.8 g

GIFT

In gratitude for your purchase of this book, I want to send you a valuable & useful GIFT!
GET YOUR GIFT

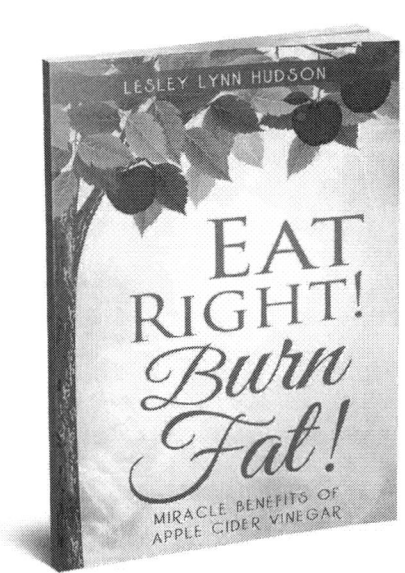

SIGN UP HERE
http://hudson.topbook.top

Do you know Apple Cider Vinegar is like magic?

Whether you want to lose some weight, fight against cancer, use it as a detox or relieve the symptoms of dozens of medical conditions, using apple cider vinegar is something you should try. And with lots of recipes included, you can also get your family taking this amazing supplement without them even knowing about it.

Read **EAT RIGHT! BURN FAT! Miracle Benefits of Apple Cider Vinegar** now and see how it can help you!

I want to pay you thanks for purchasing this book. I hope this book has provided you with some great vegan air-fried recipes which you can make easily without too much time or effort.

Could you do a small 2 min favor, please? I can't do a business without reviews, as Amazon thrives on them. It's important to me that you leave a tiny review of The Vegan Air Fryer Cookbook. Please scan the QR code with your Smartphone to be taken directly to Amazon places where you can leave a review.

or follow the link **http://www.amazon.com/ryp**

If you have any critical remarks and recommendations, send it to my email **LesleyLynnHudson@gmail.com**. This will help me make the book better thanks to you.

With great respect and appreciation,
Lesley Lynn Hudson
My email - LesleyLynnHudson@gmail.com

Made in the USA
Lexington, KY
20 November 2018